Bringing *Sexy* Back

Transform the body you have into the body you want

Pieter De Wet, M.D.

Bringing Sexy Back

Transform the body you have into the body you want

Copyright © 2012 by Pieter De Wet, M.D.

All rights reserved.
No part of this book may be reproduced or transmitted in any form or by any means
without written permission from the author.

Published by BEXSI Publishing
www.iwrotethebookonit.com

The opinions expressed by the author are not necessarily those of Bexsi Publishing, LLC. This book is designed to provide accurate and authoritative information with regard to the subject matter covered. This information is given with the understanding that neither the author nor Bexsi Publishing, LLC is engaged in rendering legal, professional advice. Since the details of your situation are fact dependent, you should additionally seek the services of a competent professional.

**Quantum Healing Institute &
Tyler Total Wellness Center
212 Old Grande Blvd., Ste C114
Tyler, Texas 75703**

Direct: 903.939.2069
Toll Free: 877.484.9735
Email: info@QHIWellness.com
http://www.qhiwellness.com

MEDICAL ADVICE DISCLAIMER

THE AUTHOR PROVIDES THE BOOK IN ITS ENTIRETY, INCLUDING ITS CONTENT, SERVICES AND DATA (collectively, "Information") CONTAINED THEREIN, AND ONLY FOR THE PURPOSES OF INFORMATION. NO MEDICAL ADVICE IS PROVIDED IN THIS BOOK, AND THE INFORMATION SHOULD NOT BE USED OR UNDERSTOOD TO BE MEDICAL ADVICE. No aspect of use of the book constitutes a patient-physician relationship between you and the Author. This includes use of, reading the book, accessing and/or browsing the website, and/or providing any information to the Author. Nothing contained in the book is intended to take the place of or substitute for the services of a licensed, trained physician or health professional licensed in your state. Nothing in this book or on the website should be relied upon for making personal health decisions. A physician licensed in your state should be used for advice and consultation in all matters relating to your health. By use of this book and website you agree that you shall not make any health or medical related decision based in whole or in part on anything contained in the Site.

Acknowledgements

I would like to acknowledge the following people who have inspired me on the journey that has led to the writing of this book. Some of them have been my teachers, some of them have been there with their support and love, and others have been a great inspiration to me as I have followed their lives and careers.

First and foremost, I would like to express my deep gratitude to my wife Cindi, who inspires me every day as a life partner, best friend, awesome mother, and my business partner who leads by example. As a matter of fact, her 75+ pounds of weight loss that she has maintained for over 10 years unequivocally proves that people can profoundly transform their lives in all areas, including obesity. I also want to thank my seven children and the staff members at QHI Wellness for their unconditional love and support. In addition, I want to thank a series of teachers I have learned from and who inspired me throughout the years. They include: Gilbert Renaud, Ph.D.; David Holt, D.O.; Lee Cowden, MD; Claude Sabbah, MD; Ryke Hamer, MD; Dietrich Klinghardt, MD; Bruce Shelton, MD, Joe Mercola, MD, Robert Rowen, MD; David Hawkins, MD; Larry Dossey, MD; Deepak Chakra, MD; and Wayne Dyer, Ph.D.

I also want to acknowledge a number of other individuals who inspire me with their personal revolutions of improved health, including those whose stories are told in this book. I want to thank each of them for granting me permission to tell their stories. A heartfelt thanks to the following people, who have given their unconditional support to our efforts to make a difference in this world. Thanks to: Suzanne and Fanned Seidel, Ruthie Spence, Corene and Clarence Schwab, John and Vicki Yahn, and Frank Jordan.

I would like to extend a special thanks to my gracious patients; John Martin, Gary Johnson, Veronica Smith, Sal Landeros, Vicky Brannon, Brandy Lucas, and Cathy Bailey who courageously shared their stories in this book. And finally, to Susan Spence, who spent many hours to help review and edit this book for you. And above all, I acknowledge my Creator, the source of all things, including this book.

Table of Contents

Foreword……………………………………………….. 7

Preface………………………………………………..…… 12

Introduction……………………………………….. 15

Chapter 1……………………………………..………… 22
Why Everything You Know about Obesity is Wrong

Chapter 2…………………………………………....… 43
Your Grandmother Made You Fat: Epigenetics

Chapter 3……………………………………..……… 92
Turning Your Metabolism into a Nuclear Reactor

Chapter 4……………………………………………....…112
A Layman's Guide to a Doctor's World: Understanding Fat Physiology

Chapter 5……………………………………..………131
Body Rehab: Removing Obstacles for Great Metabolism

Chapter 6……………………………………..………153
Lifestyle: Time to Release the Fat and MOVE

Chapter 7……………………………………..………201
Spiritual Fat: The Final Conflict

Bibliography……………………………………..……..226

Foreword

This past summer I had the pleasure of meeting Dr. Pieter De Wet. I was in his office and noticed the material about weight loss that was at the front desk. It suggested that I could lose as much as 40 pounds in 40 days. I immediately inquired about the program, and within a week I was in Dr. De Wet's office starting his version of the β HCG Weight Loss program. My starting weight was 293 lbs. I went through a myriad of tests which included blood work, an EKG, and a sleep test because of my morbid obesity and grave concerns about possible complications from my weight.

Prior to this testing, I had always felt like I was in good health in spite of my weight. My blood pressure was normal, and I had high energy. But, I was surprised to discover after not having been to a doctor in years, that my body was beginning to deteriorate. My blood pressure, while not incredibly alarming, was higher than it had ever been, and the numbers for liver blood tests, cholesterol, and triglycerides, etc. were extremely elevated. Dr. De Wet was particularly alarmed at the liver numbers as they were twice the norm. He was concerned about a possible cirrhosis of the liver. There were several supplements that he recommended for me along with the β HCG as part of his unique weight loss program, which I took.

I went home that day feeling energized and excited. I read through the instructions word for word and nearly memorized how to move forward. I even got to pig out for two days ahead of time, which I thought would be really cool and guilt free. (Actually, it was difficult to do) Eating everything in sight for two days is not easy at all. It felt like there was a psychological reason for doing this, even over and above the medical reasons, and that was to create an aversion to fatty, sugary, starchy, and processed foods in order to help move me along at the beginning.

After these initial fat-loading days, I was supposed to cut my calorie intake to 500 calories per day, choosing from very specific food options that are laid out in great detail in Dr. De Wet's instruction manual. In order to make it easy on me, my wife essentially made my meals for me ahead of time. All I needed to do was pull the food out of the freezer, warm it up (NOT in a microwave oven, to avoid the radiation), and eat. I had done many diets in the past at 1200 calories a day and virtually starved the entire time, so doing 500 calories per day was shocking to me based on my past experience. I wasn't sure how this was going to work, but I was determined to make it happen no matter how bad it appeared to be. I began the first day of gorging and rubbing the HCG cream on my forearms. I got through the first day not really wanting to eat anymore, but I had another day of gorging ahead of me. I tried to enjoy it, thinking I knew what was to come. The second day was really tough. I did not want to eat, but forced myself. When day three came, I began the 500 calorie per day restriction, and it was actually tough only because my body reacted to thinking it was going to be starved as it had many times before. I felt tired and hungry. Once I realized psychologically that my body was not going to be starved, this feeling went away and by day 4, I was rocking! When you use the β HCG, it literally is like a lock and key that gives you access to all of the pathological fat stores, enabling your body to preferentially burn as many as 4,000 calories of fat from these fat stores per day, depending on your activity levels.

Day by day, I got stronger. My body was being fed through the bloodstream off of my excess body fat. I had no hunger, I had tons of energy, and in the first week, I lost almost 17 pounds. WOW! I was pumped! Losing that much weight so quickly did, however, have one side effect. My body was already deficient in potassium and vitamin D. I started to have major muscle cramps, and because I had a bad lower back, the muscle spasms began to pull at a vertebra that was out of place, which almost incapacitated me. Dr. De Wet immediately put me on large quantities of potassium and magnesium, and the spasms slowly went away. My advice to anyone reading this is to make sure your body is not deficient in any major nutrients (like potassium or magnesium) when you start this program, because losing weight rapidly like this can accentuate these deficiencies. I strongly recommend that if you are going to do a program such as β HCG, ONLY do it in consultation with someone who is very knowledgeable, to prevent complications. I advanced very quickly through the rest of the 42 day program and lost a total of 48 pounds. I have never experienced anything like it. It made me more and more excited about getting to my goal of 100 pounds lost. It is important to note that I far exceeded expectations, I'm happy to say, because as I found out subsequently, the average weight loss for a man is 31 pounds per cycle and 22 pounds per cycle for a woman. This means I lost a lot of fluid weight initially, which was the reason why my body became deficient in electrolytes.

Towards the end of my first cycle of the program, I began to get concerned about the 6 week break you must take in order to keep the body from becoming immune to the HCG. I had been told by friends that I was going to just gain it right back, however, I read in the instruction manual that this would not happen as long as I followed the directions to stay away from breads, sugars, and grains during that time. I am very proud to say that during that time I actually lost another 5 pounds and, for the most part, enjoyed eating normally again.

I must tell you about another very exciting thing that I experienced at the end of the first cycle. Dr. De Wet suggested that I take another round of blood panels in order to make sure the elevated numbers that were so alarming in the beginning were coming down properly. If they weren't, we would need to attack the problem from another direction. I remember the day very well when I found out the results. Live on the air on Dr. De Wet's radio program, he informed me that every single elevated number, including my very alarming liver number, was perfectly normal.

48 pounds in 42 days…incredible!

I still am amazed at how the β HCG, along with certain supplements, gave my body the opportunity to heal itself so quickly.

I finally began my second cycle on the program. I was so excited, but at the time was a bit sad that I would have to go through Thanksgiving and Christmas (my favorite time of the year) without being able to eat everything I wanted. I made a decision at my 70th pound lost (in just 100 days!) that I was going to suspend the cycle 2 weeks early in order to enjoy the holidays—kind of as a reward for my own success. I was able to enjoy the holidays guilt-free, and while I did gain a few pounds, I was not worried in the least because I had found a miracle! I'm now in round three and working on the last 30 pounds of my goal.

I was on my way to having a major heart attack, but probably the best thing overall is that I have a totally different quality of life. I don't run into door jambs, I don't need a seatbelt extension on airplanes, I don't get out of breath just walking through the house, I can sleep, I can pick things up off the floor without any issue—the list goes on and on.

My heartfelt thanks to Dr. Pieter De Wet, Cindi De Wet, and the entire staff at QHI Wellness—my new HEROES and friends!

In my opinion, Dr. De Wet saved my life.

—John Martin

Preface

This book is, first and foremost, inspired by my own experience. Like so many others, I have been inflicted by problems with excessive weight, which have plagued me ever since I started going to medical school. I had other events occur in my life that contributed to further weight gain. Even from the very beginning, I had a feeling that my weight gain was not just because of how many calories I was consuming or my lack of physical activity. I had a very deep sense that my emotions also had something to do with it. Although I couldn't figure out how to resolve some of these conflicts, my intuition told me that resolving the emotional conflicts within me were the key to a permanent solution for not only my extra weight, but the obesity of a nation.

The book is inspired from the fact that we're dealing with an extraordinary epidemic in our society of obesity and other chronic illnesses associated with obesity—not just obesity itself, but also the way people look at themselves. There is a crisis of self-confidence that so many people have.

The goal of this book is to change the way people look at themselves, whether they're obese or not, so they can see the beauty in everything. There's an inherent beauty in each human being that is critical for us to see if we want to battle the prevalent misery plaguing our society. The issue of obesity includes not just the physical health implications of being overweight, but the mental, emotional, social, and spiritual implications of how we perceive ourselves. The title of this book is inspired by the idea that we want to look at things in a different light. We want to not just lose weight and regain health, but we want to teach people to start their process to deeply and profoundly learn to love and accept themselves. This book is about how to achieve and enjoy the body that you want, which doesn't necessarily mean that you have to lose a lot of weight. Achieving and enjoying the body that you want starts with accepting and loving the body that you have.

The most critical difference between this book and so many other books on obesity, weight loss, improving aesthetics, and so forth is the premise. The premise of this book is to teach people to change their minds as to the way they look at themselves. It is possible to transform one's health in profound ways. Surely many of people desire to lose weight, improve our appearance, etc. But in order to do that it is absolutely critical that the premise be changed. A large part of this book is focused on how obesity is a survival program instead of a health problem. If obesity is actually helping us increase our chances of survival, then it can and should be perceived as something we should be eternally thankful for.

The other premise of this book is to help people embrace an attitude of gratitude for every aspect of their appearance, personality, habits and even their addictions.

What you will learn is that we have a program running that defines the exact weight we are, at a given moment. That program has to be discovered, changed and resolved in order for us to have the long-term success in achieving the bodies we want. We'll also discuss the physiological, hormonal, dietary, and exercise aspects, but from a perspective of individualizing. This book is about each person discovering his or her own optimal diet, exercise and sleep patterns. We also indulge a little bit in the concepts of cleaning the body out and realizing that fat is there for a purpose and in order to clear fat, we have to detox what is released from the fat when it starts melting away. We also uncover innovative methods to facilitate the weight loss process (for example, the β HCG weight loss program). β HCG is a system I have personally used for my own health and has contributed to tremendous success in my own healing process and to literally hundreds of other people. We have assembled some stories to inspire others who are affected, not just with weight issues, but with other health issues that literally have warped the person's self-image.

My goal for you, after you read this book from the beginning to the end, is to have a brand new appreciation for the habits that promote excessive weight. You will not only learn to love yourself unconditionally, but love your weight, obesity, or overweight issues and even your habits. The paradox is if you want to reform your health or your weight, it is critical to start with deep and profound self-acceptance and self-love.

Introduction

When you pick up this book, many of you are probably wondering why a book would be called *Bringing Sexy Back: Transform the Body You Have into the Body You Want*. Most people don't see themselves as sexy, beautiful, attractive, or special. In other words, they feel unattractive physically and also look at themselves in a negative light from an emotional, mental, relational, and spiritual perspective. Most people compare themselves to others and feel like they fall short. But, when we use others as the benchmark to compare ourselves against, we will never feel good about ourselves. We are all individuals with our own views on what constitutes beauty. In fact, beauty is a fleeting concept that has changed drastically over the centuries. For example, when we go back and look at the paintings of the famous Dutch artist Rembrandt, we see that his subjects included naked women who were very voluptuous and curvy. When you look at today's standards, these women would be classified as moderately overweight or in some cases even obese, and yet, in their day, they were seen as the symbol of rapturous beauty. Back then the thin women who graced the covers of *Cosmopolitan* or *Playboy* today would be considered sickly or even anorexic.

It's simply a matter of how you frame beauty. Right now most people equate being extremely thin with being beautiful, but even that is shifting. Women are getting fed up with society seeing them as ugly because of skewed media definitions of so-called beauty. We all want to be beautiful, and we all can reframe ourselves as beautiful, even if our body weight and body shape doesn't necessarily match perfectly what's in vogue at any given moment.

Whether we are underweight or obese, it is critical that we learn to reframe the way we see ourselves. Every one of us has an element of sexiness. There are elements of beauty and attractiveness that already exist in each of us, and they are much more than skin deep. Reframing the way we see beauty is about understanding the deeper meaning behind every single curve or fat pad on our bodies—therefore, the *perfection* of what *is*.

You have the ability to achieve the body you want and to truly enjoy it. Some people achieve the bodies they want but feel miserable about it because they have to starve themselves to maintain it. Is that how we define *sexy*? Certainly not. I think we would all agree that being sexy isn't just about looking great: it's also about feeling great inside your skin. There is something appealing about someone who is confident and truly enjoys their body, no matter what it looks like. In the end, sexiness is not about what your body looks like, but in how you feel about your body and inside your skin. Enjoying your body is critical to achieving and maintaining a high level of health no matter what your body looks like, and this doesn't just apply to your weight, but also to your body shape. Learning to love your body and enjoy it is essential to overcoming not just obesity, but any type of illness.

I believe that the key to healing obesity, like with all diseases, lies first and foremost in reframing how we look at it. In other words, we have to see it for what it is. My work in holistic medicine has taught me the power that conflict resolution has for everyone. Disease is a biological solution to an emotional or biological dilemma—not an inexplicable curse that comes out of nowhere to torment us endlessly. As you read this book, you will understand exactly what I mean by this. I've seen so many amazing transformations of people who have defied the odds and reversed the so-called irreversible, including morbid obesity and all its associated afflictions, such as diabetes and hypertension. These are people for whom things appeared hopeless and for whom the only hope had become radical treatments such as gastric bypass surgery. I will be sharing some of the stories of these individuals with you with explanations of how they transcended their limitations and succeeded against all odds in transforming their health. The key to curing obesity lies in discovering and clearing the conflict(s) that lie at the root of the condition.

In this book, we will often refer to a treatment modality called Recall Healing or recall therapy. The science of Recall Healing applies not just to obesity but also to cancer, diabetes, and virtually any other health problem imaginable. This book will help you to look at not just obesity differently, but also all the associated health problems with being overweight. We have been taught by those in the medical profession that obesity is behind numerous other epidemics of chronic illnesses. That stems at least in part from erroneous conclusions, primarily because we are not looking deep enough to realize that every illness has its own unique associated biological conflict that programs for it. Even though there are some common denominators between obesity and these other health problems, the source of these issues is nearly always traceable to an unresolved emotional conflict.

The more we learn about Recall Healing and how our body becomes programmed for specific diseases, the more we discover that every disease is a separate and unique biological program. This is why it is possible to weigh 500 pounds and *not* have hypertension or diabetes, for example. On the other hand, someone can be at so-called normal body weight and suffer from all of the health problems usually associated with the obese. You may have a greater chance of suffering from these types of health problems if you are overweight, but in the end, it does not mean if you are obese you automatically develop some of these so-called complications.

I had to learn this principle the hard way in medical school. I remember seeing patients who had been treated for cancer with chemotherapy and drugs. Right before my eyes, they would go from looking fairly healthy to being frail and sick-looking. Their hair gone, with swollen faces and bodies, they looked and acted more ill than when they came in. I kept asking whether sometimes the drugs used to treat these diseases could be worse than the disease itself. Of course, that was the 'conventional' way, to do everything possible to get rid of the cancer. Many nights I went home after my hospital rounds, feeling frustrated and aggravated by everything I saw. I didn't see the whole picture yet.

I believed traditional medicine seemed to have solutions for many illnesses and it was good at saving lives and crisis management. At that time, I thought conventional medicine had its place, so I practiced integrated medicine, using both alternative and conventional treatments. I saw many cases where conventional medicine was amazing, especially as a young doctor, working in the emergency room.

However, at the end of the day I was not satisfied. I knew there had to be more to this thing called medicine. The solution to any health problem should not make us *sicker*. It should not cause us to wonder if the treatment is worse than the illness. True healing is about treating the whole person and the root cause of the health problems that lie within. This book will help you understand the conflicts you face and how they are responsible for your obesity. When you start to realize these conflicts, you can then name them, deal with them, and get rid of them as easily as discarding a piece of paper.

The body never does anything without purpose and meaning. Every piece of biology is always in alignment with the deeper subconscious, and it is in some way a conflict manifestation. Sometimes the conflict is from my own life, and sometimes it is something that happened while I was in the womb, such as a conflict my parents acquired. A fetus often takes on the conflict of the parents like a sponge because the baby does not have its own identity until it is about a year old when the baby starts developing a sense of individual identity. Up until that point, the baby cannot differentiate between itself and its parents. All the unresolved emotional or psychological conflicts of the parent become a biological conflict for the child and plays out in the child's biology either physically or emotionally.

The third element is the genealogical download, so sometimes if you can't find something in your own life, then you know that it is genealogical and carried epigenetically and is manifesting as a result of something that happened to someone in your past.

When we understand how our bodies work and why we struggle so much with our weight, we can start to see the beauty that exists in ourselves. It doesn't matter how much fat you've accumulated. It doesn't matter if you're underweight or suffering from an eating disorder. There is a purpose for every speck of fat on your body. It's there for a reason, and we all have the ability to work with our bodies to uncover that reason.

You have the ability to achieve the body you want and truly enjoy it. Some people achieve the bodies they want but feel miserable about it because they have to starve themselves in order to maintain it.

Is that sexy?

Certainly not! I think we would all agree that being sexy is not just about looking great: it's also about feeling great inside the skin you're in. There's something appealing about someone who is confident and truly enjoys their body—no matter what it looks like. In the end, the sexiness lies not in the way their body looks, but in how they feel inside of that body.

Enjoying your body is critical to achieving and maintaining a high level of health, no matter what your body looks like, and this doesn't just apply to your weight. Enjoyment of your body is essential to battling every kind of disease, including obesity.

That should include enjoying how you look, how you move and the physicality of relationships. In order to open up in your relationships with others, you must love, accept and enjoy who you are first, not the other way around.

Chapter One:

Why Everything You Know about Obesity is *Wrong*

"Obesity is the body's solution to a deeper conflict. Resolve the conflict and you release the obesity."

—Dr. Pieter De Wet

Obesity is a problem that has plagued our society for centuries. Many people and highly respected professionals believe they know the truth about obesity. However, there are hidden root causes and belief systems that are seriously flawed. "Just exercise and eat the right foods, and you'll be a healthy weight," common sense dictates.

Maybe not.

Many people fail to lose weight because they don't understand how the body works or how the mind and the emotional and spiritual realms work with the body. They also don't realize that obesity occurs as a *result* of these realms colliding with each other. In fact, we should be thankful for obesity because it is actually the body's solution to a deeper dilemma that's not just physical, but also emotional, mental, relational, and spiritual as well.

Emotional Reasons for Obesity

Obesity is a biological program launched by the brain to respond to a deeper conflict or unresolved emotional stress that threatens to overwhelm consciousness. In this context, we see the body as a container, and obesity as a biological program. This program is launched by the brain in response to deeper conflicts or unresolved emotional stressors that threaten to overwhelm consciousness. The brain then downloads to a small portion of itself and to the body. As Claude Sabbah once said, "Disease is the brain's best solution to keep the person alive as long as possible. Thus, disease is a survival program."

The brain has to resolve stress somehow when it is overwhelmingly threatened, so it downloads the stress to a smaller part of itself and to the body at the same time. There is also always a connection between the type of stress and the specific disease that manifests in the specific organ. For example, if someone develops breast cancer, we know that there is some kind of a nesting conflict, especially if the cancer is either one of the two most common types (adenocarcinoma or ductal carcinoma). This is why it affects women more than 20 times more often than men, and not just because women have bigger breasts. Both women and men can get breast cancer, but women are more likely to develop it because they are far more likely to develop what we call "conflicts of the nest." The conflict of the nest tends to be associated with issues related to the family (i.e., children, spouse, parents), home, or even domestic animals or a business.

Men, on the other hand, tend to deal with these same types of issues differently and are more likely to take them on as, for example, territorial conflicts. Coronary artery disease, which is much more prevalent in men, especially in middle aged groups, is usually related to conflict of lost territory or the threatened loss of territory. For a man, losing his house may program for a heart attack, whereas for a woman, losing the same house may program for breast cancer.

A woman develops breast cancer because of what's happening in her nest environment. For example, if she loses her child or her child becomes seriously ill or is severely injured in an accident, then her brain will automatically be threatened with overwhelming stress. It will automatically download that stress to a smaller part of the brain that is associated with the organ that is most congruent with the conflict, which would be the breast. Then it will also download to the breast itself, which then becomes the container for that conflict. The threatened loss of a child is the biological invariant that can manifest as breast cancer. The biological invariant refers to a specific disease caused by a specific conflict. Until the brain is able to deal with what is going on and get rid of the conflict, it will be held in that smaller part of the brain and in the breast.

If there's a likelihood that the conflict will continue to overwhelm her consciousness if it is brought back, the brain will keep it contained in the smaller part of the brain and in the organ itself. However, the moment we become capable of dealing with the stress and bring it back to consciousness, not only does the conflict clear from our consciousness, but the physical manifestations in the brain and the breast will also disappear.

Dealing with obesity is about more than simply taking in fewer calories than what you use during the day. That, of course, is an over-simplified perspective. There is some truth to the fact that the more we eat, the more likely we are to be suffering from obesity. The calorie intake does not equate to anywhere near a 100 percent correlation between calorie intake and obesity. We know this because many people have very fast burning metabolisms and can eat as much as they want and never have problems with obesity. Others eat very few calories, and yet they cannot budge their body weight in any way, shape, or form, especially not downward.

There are many different factors that contribute to being overweight or obese, and they all need to be taken into account if we want to find a permanent solution for being overweight. It's much more than simple physiology, which tells us which tissues in the body are not working properly but doesn't tell us anything about the cause of the dysfunction. Obesity is directly connected with the functions of the organs, hormones, detox systems, and the brain. Obesity is also connected to calorie intake, food choices and food quality. It is important to remember that diseases like obesity occur because of the brain and body's response to deeper conflicts. These deeper conflicts affect not only the brain, but physiology. They affect the function of organs, levels of certain hormones, and the speed of metabolism.

In order to heal a disease, we have to discover and clear it at its source. The source can be on any one of five levels. In my first book, *Heal Thyself: Transform your Life, Transform your Health,* I have a chapter on the five levels of healing that discusses this in great detail. For example, in treating obesity, it is critical for us to discover the source of the disease. The source is rarely at the physical body level and is almost always to be found in the mental body, the intuitive body, or the spirit body. However, this does not negate the impact of physical aspects you may have such calorie intake, food choices, toxins in your food, or the effect of electromagnetic fields on your energy body. We are not a meat suit with a brain. Our bodies have five distinct levels that interconnect at all times.

The five levels of our body are:

1. Physical body

2. Energy body

3. Mental body

4. Intuitive body

5. Spirit body

Think of illness as a three-stage rocket. At the top of the rocket is the psyche, which includes all of our emotions, thoughts, decisions, feelings, beliefs, religious backgrounds, education, and conditioning. In other words, the psyche can also be described as the way we resolve our daily problems.

The second stage of the three-stage rocket is what we call the automatic brain, which is the part that is focused on physical survival from moment to moment. The automatic brain implements its program through the autonomic nervous system. The automatic brain is never wrong: it simply takes information from the psyche and when the psyche is overwhelmed it downloads the conflict into the automatic brain.

The third stage of this rocket occurs when the automatic brain downloads the conflict through the autonomic nervous system into the body. The automatic brain also downloads unresolved conflicts to the brain tissue itself. The body and the brain are controlled by the automatic brain through the autonomic nervous system. That's how all diseases, including obesity, occur in the first place.

Physical Manifestations of Your Thoughts and Beliefs

Let's take a look at how obesity develops from the perspective outlined above. Fat tissue in the human body is controlled by a certain part of the brain called the cerebellum, which sits behind and on top of the brain stem. It is located below the cerebrum, which is the bigger part of the brain that controls conscious thought and fine movement in the body. The cerebellum is the part of the brain that controls fine movement and coordination of movement. It is also associated with the reflexes that allow us to withdraw from threats automatically without conscious thought. The logical conclusion, therefore, is fat is often created in the human body for protection from outside threats.

There is another part of the brain that is involved with fat metabolism—the hypothalamus. The hypothalamus is the critical control center in the brain that controls hormone production in the body, as well as fat metabolism and appetite. Certain types of psychological conflicts, when threatening to overwhelm consciousness, will be downloaded to this part of the brain.

Whenever we experience a conflict that programs our body for obesity, the cerebellum and the hypothalamus are intimately involved. In order to understand obesity, we need to understand what the body uses fat for. Fat is the body's most efficient way of storing calories. Fat is also the best insulator the body has against cold, and fat is lighter than water which can be critical in saving one's life in the water. Fat naturally creates physical padding against attack. In the next few paragraphs we will explore some of the conflict programming behind obesity.

- Obesity can be a form of protection against drowning because having excessive fat makes it easier to float. If you had an episode of near-drowning, for example, in life, or even if one of your ancestors actually drowned or had a massive trauma that led to a near drowning, there is very likely to be a program of conflict in the family that relates to this trauma of drowning. In other words, obesity can be a physical manifestation of what happened in the past and what your biology has put in place to reduce your likelihood of drowning. If that conflict is never fully cleared, spoken about, or brought to consciousness, then it will be passed down from generation to generation until someone becomes aware of it or until it spontaneously washes out of the genealogical tree which tends to happen after a certain number of generations.

- Obesity can be a form of protection against starvation. For example, if you nearly died from starvation as a child, like in the case of a child who develops severe dysentery and nearly dies, it is very possible that the child will develop obesity later on in their life as a response to any kind of stress because of that original starvation program. This also has a generational implication. For example, if you had an ancestor or ancestors who died of starvation, for instance, three generations ago, there is more likely to be obesity in the downstream generations as a result. It's like a subconscious biological program that literally has the biological purpose to protect others in the family against starvation by storing more calories in the form of fat. We typically do not find a conscious memory of this, but it certainly is present in the subconscious, especially when the drama occurred during the life of the person who is afflicted with this problem. From a generational perspective, it comes through as a epigenetic imprint, which we will discuss later in this book.

- Obesity can be a physical manifestation of the response to previous attacks in the family. An attack can be real, imaginary, virtual, or symbolic. For example, if a child grows up in a home with parents who fight all the time, he might wish in his subconscious mind to be bigger so that he is able to stand up to the parent who is causing the fight or can get between the parents to get them to stop fighting. If a father abuses a mother, for example, the child's subconscious brain will set off a biological program to start increasing the size of the body of that child. The body will often develop an extra layer of fat because the brain is programmed to launch that kind of protective mechanism in the body.

- Obesity can also be related to neglect or abandonment. Again, it can be real, imaginary, virtual, or symbolic. For instance, a person who grows up and was emotionally neglected compared to his or her siblings will often gain weight. It's almost like the body is saying on behalf of that person, "Hey, notice me. I'm important, too." The body becomes fatter, the person can stand out and be more visible to the neglectful parent or parents.

- Obesity can also be a way for the body to deal with the experience of a loss. For example, a woman who loses a baby that was about six pounds will often gain six pounds immediately upon the loss of the baby or maintain six pounds after the pregnancy to symbolize the loss that she suffered. In a way, her subconscious mind just cannot get past that loss. The baby is symbolically stored in her body until the loss is fully processed, which often never happens unless someone becomes aware of this connection.

Another way to appreciate the programming for obesity is to look at extreme opposites. For instance, if someone suffers from anorexia nervosa, the traumas and beliefs tend to be the opposite of those suffered by someone with obesity. For example, one of my patients was the third child in a family with two older siblings who were quite a bit older than her. Their father was extremely abusive towards the older children, so when she was born, her biological program was to be as small and unobtrusive as possible so that she did not become a target of her aggressive father.

At a biological level, she did not want to become a victim of the abuse, so her brain programmed her body to become as small as possible so that she could literally disappear in the cracks of the walls so that her father would not notice her and turn his violence upon her. The father, being an alcoholic, used to come home and pick fights with the older children and their mother. My patient managed to escape the abuse by staying in her room and acting as unobtrusively as possible. Later on in her life, she developed severe anorexia nervosa, which started shortly after her parents got divorced. She was 16 years old. The stress of the divorce literally set off this program that was already part of her biology and cleared up when she became clearly aware of and was able to transcend the conflict she had stored in her subconscious.

Among other things, she had to learn to forgive her father for his actions towards them and their mother when she and her siblings were younger. She forgave him by gaining insight into her own childhood traumas and by understanding *his* childhood traumas, (which were considerable) and also by understanding the genealogical programming on both her father's and her mother's side. She had to forgive not only her father, but her mother, who chose to stay with this abusive man and who did not protect her or the other children against their father. She was able to forgive both her father and her mother completely. Shortly thereafter, her body began to normalize to a healthy weight.

In a similar way when you discover the conflicts that program for your obesity it becomes easier to resolve this long-term or even permanently. Oftentimes your obesity will literally disappear like magic, even without a specific focus on diet, cutting calories, or exercise. This is the magic potential of Recall Healing.

Achieve Optimal Health by Changing Your Thoughts

In order to heal from an affliction like obesity, it is critical for us to learn to change our thoughts. In order to change our thoughts, however, we need to realize that thoughts follow beliefs. In other words, to change our thoughts, we have to evaluate and change our beliefs. Basically, you're as healthy as the beliefs you hold in your mind and the emotions and feelings that are generated as a consequence of those beliefs. For instance, if you tend to be a person with very negative and self-defeating beliefs, then your health will be rather poor as a result. However, positive beliefs lead to preponderance of positive emotions, which are more likely to be conducive to healing.

This is a very elementary description of the roles that emotions and beliefs play in our overall health. However, it is indisputable that negative emotions contribute to disease, yet are part and parcel of everyday life. It's impossible to live without emotional conflicts because they serve as road signs on the highway of life. They come up when we are going in a direction that is counterproductive or self-destructive. On the other hand, positive emotions are like road signs that tell us that we are going in a direction that is constructive and uplifting. Becoming aware of our emotions and underlying beliefs are critical parts of healing.

Pain and negative emotions are critical for healing because they remind us of what is broken or out of balance within us, either within our bodies or within our thoughts. Emotional and physical pain go hand in hand and help us to redirect our lives and keep us on the right path.

If you are struggling with your weight, you may want to take a closer look at the following two myths and how they might be contributing to your affliction.

Myth #1: "I am fat because of heredity."

Many people believe they are obese because they believe that they inherited a genetic code for obesity. They see obesity in other members of their family, so it's quite natural for them to believe that this has been genetically preordained. This faulty belief system will prevent a lot of people from losing weight and keeping it off. When we change this belief system by realizing that the obesity is a *programmed* condition and this programming is rarely due to genetics, a turning point is reached. Once the belief begins to shift, it can be influenced much more readily, creating an easier path to overcome obesity. Believing that obesity is genetically based is counterproductive. Our emotions and even the experiences of our ancestors impact on how our genes express themselves creates a much more empowering belief system that allows us the space to change that expression. This critical insight helps us create a much more empowering belief system that allows us the space to even change that expression of our genetic code. In short, even if there are generations of overweight parents and grandparents, it is within our power to break the cycle through a change in our beliefs, thoughts, emotions, and actions today. The field of science that studies the factors that affect the expression of our genetic code is called epigenetics.

Myth #2: "The right diet will make me lose weight."

Most people believe that they are eating healthy even when they are not. When it comes to nutrition a lot of people have dysfunctional belief systems about what is healthy and what is not. For instance, if you believe that margarine is healthy to eat, as people have been taught to believe for the last 30 years or more, it will make it nearly impossible for you to lose weight. If you believe the food pyramid, which has been promoted as the symbol for healthy eating by the USDA for the last three or four decades, then you will also have a very hard time losing weight and maintaining a healthy body weight. Another faulty belief is the common misconception that eating foods with artificial sweeteners in them will help you lose weight. The reality is artificial sweeteners do very little to help us lose weight or even to maintain a healthy weight.

It's not always possible to figure out what is true and what is not through based on what we are taught by the medical establishment, the media, and our government entities. We are fed a lot of myths by popular culture, outright lies by special interest groups, and misinformation by irresponsible marketers. Most of these powerful groups have great influence on the media because of their paid advertising and political clout. We also receive a lot of misinformation from our governmental health agencies as well. The bottom line is we all need to learn to listen to our intuition when it comes to figuring out right from wrong. We need to learn to question every so-called truth spread by the media and the conventional medical community.

We need to listen to our bodies.

Another key to changing your thoughts is to change or shift your mindset. A lot of people think of themselves as physically challenged (handicapped), and as a consequence of this belief system, they minimize their exertion. They think because of their label, they somehow are not capable of doing much at all of a physical nature. As a result, we have an ever-growing number of *invalids* all vying for the handicapped zones around town. The result of this mindset creates another limit on the potential long-term success of weight loss.

In order to be successful with weight loss, we have to literally reframe who we are and how we see ourselves. Even the most physically challenged human being can inspire us with what they are capable of doing in spite of their handicap. For example, one of my clients I've been working with and who has been following my β HCG weight loss program over the internet (www.shopqhi.com) has been in a wheelchair since his early 20s and is now in his 50s. He has lost over 60 pounds over a period of about three and a half months. One of the mental strategies he used was to refuse to see himself as handicapped. He gets out of his house and goes about his business every day and gets regular exercise. He has every incentive and opportunity to park as close as possible to the door of any establishment.

Instead, with the intent of getting exercise, he goes against the grain and believes he deserves no special treatment. He lives a very active lifestyle for a man who is in a wheelchair. Paralyzed from the waist down he continues to experience great success with his overall health, weight loss, as a businessman and a family man.

His beliefs inspires thousands of others around him.

When we begin to see ourselves in a different light—seeing ourselves as infinitely capable, even of the impossible—we can begin the process of successful weight loss and weight maintenance. It just takes a change of mindset, including about what is framed as fun and what is not. A lot of people have very rigid belief systems about what is enjoyable and what isn't. There are a lot of people who hate exercise and feel like they are torturing themselves every time they work out, while others love to exercise. Anyone can change their mindsets by looking at things in a different light.

Gary's Story

Gary Johnson came to see me three weeks after talking to me on the phone. He has accomplished extraordinary feats since then with his health. He's lost a total of 57 pounds between November 2010 and August 2011. He has gotten off all of the drugs he used for diabetes and his blood pressure medicines within three days of first seeing me in Texas. His diabetes symptoms and signs were gone, including his elevated blood sugars, along with his sleep apnea and hypertension in 72 hours. His osteoarthritis symptoms, including his knees, were 75 percent better, and all symptoms of gall bladder disease were reversed. His chronic fatigue was resolved, his high cholesterol improved, and his high triglycerides reversed when checked soon after that first visit. His elevated liver enzymes were markedly improved, and his energy was up to 100 percent better. In other words, Gary received a new lease on life and a massive emotional and spiritual shift, to boot. He also conquered a lot of negative emotions, including conflicts linked to his work, his profession, and conflicts of devaluation he has struggled with for most of his life.

That's not the way he started.

Like many people, his ideas about weight loss were nearly all wrong. He desperately wanted to *Bring Sexy Back* in his life.

"I was a wreck. Prior to meeting Dr. De Wet, I was overweight, out of shape and had descended into rather poor health. I am not sure how I ended up with chronic fatigue, overweight and totally 'un-sexy' but I was at a loss. I had tried some fad diets and exercise, but nothing had worked.

I was about to give up.

On December 14, 2010, I was flipping around on my satellite radio looking for a Christian radio station to listen to and ended up listening to Dr. De Wet's show, on Family Talk Radio-Sirius XM Satellite Radio (The show is called "Dr. Pieter De Wet Live on Toginet.com"). The next day he was on again, and I became so intrigued that I started thinking that I should give him a call. I had a phone conversation with his staff and told them what I was going through. They scheduled me an appointment for an educational consult for me with Dr. De Wet.

I actually started getting sick a week before Thanksgiving, and I got caught up in what I call the "conventional medical system." I went to my regular doctor and had an ultrasound and then a series of tests that eventually ended in another ultrasound. My doctor sent me to a surgeon, telling me that my gall bladder had to come out. The surgeon said he did not think that was necessary and that my pancreas was inflamed and my liver was not functioning properly. All of those tests ended up costing about $50,000, and I still did not have a solution.

When I called Dr. De Wet's office, after discussing all options, I decided to hold off on the surgery until I could see him. Dr. Dr. Wet told me to go on a modified fast, and I lost 14 pounds between December 14th and December 27th.

I went to see Dr. De Wet on December 26, 2010, and I saw him four days in a row to work on my health. At the time I was a diabetic, and I had been on insulin and other diabetic medicines. One of the medications I was on has been shown to cause inflammation of the pancreas. At my first appointment with Dr. De Wet, he told me to stop taking my diabetic medicines. I stopped taking all of them, and the miraculous thing was when I came back home, as of December 30th, I had no blood sugar problems. I took my blood sugar on the 30th, and it was 90. I thought it was a mistake, so I took it again and got the same result. I went down to the store and bought a new blood sugar monitor because I thought that my other one must have been broken, but I got the same result. I had been off my insulin and diabetic meds for four days at that point, and my blood sugar was perfect. Since then I have not had any more *blood sugar problems.*

My overall health is remarkable.

Every time I come back from seeing Dr. De Wet, everyone at my office remarks at how much healthier I look. It was incredible to hear that after my very first visit with him. People who saw me every day knew right away that I looked different—a whole lot better than I had been in a long time.

By this point, I am no longer tired, and I always follow the program that Dr. De Wet gave me to the best of my ability. One of the best parts of my treatment from Dr. De Wet was the Recall Healing, which has been very instrumental in helping me come to grips with the unresolved conflicts affecting my life. I've been getting these unresolved wounds healed and out of my life.

What's great about Dr. De Wet's program is that it is all about whole health and weight loss. All the physical things are there to help you, and he is with you every step of the way. He wants to see you succeed and knows that his methods are tried and true.

When I first called Dr. De Wet, I was very skeptical. That Christmas, the night before my appointment, I was wondering if I really wanted to go, and in the back of my mind, a voice said, 'Go.' I started out being the most skeptical person, not looking for anything to come out of this, and it totally changed my life, not just from a medical standpoint, but also in terms of my entire life. Very few things in life can have such a dramatic change and impact in your life, changing how you look at things, the way you deal with things, and how you handle your health and medical decisions.

A short time ago I received a certified letter from my previous doctor, who was firing me as a patient because I was not following his advice. But now my health is extremely good. I feel at peace and much calmer than I had ever been. I'm not taking any medicine for my high blood pressure. The last time I went to see Dr. De Wet, he did segment therapy, which is a series of injections, in parts of my body, including my knees. What is really remarkable about this is that I have had chronic pain in both of my knees since I was 15 years old. I was a competitive athlete, and I'd had knee surgeries in the past. I lived with constant and severe pain in both of my knees. After a while, you learn to live with it, but Dr. De Wet did segment therapy on my knees, and the pain is gone. I haven't been totally pain free since I was 15 years old when I injured my knee that first time. The first time I walked on a treadmill after I received that injection in my knee, my brain was trying to locate the pain that it normally experienced. Over time, the pain does gradually come back, but it has never come back to the point where it was. I am 50 to 60 percent better on pain.

What was especially interesting about the Recall Healing was the fact that I had always wanted to be a professional baseball player. When I was 15, I prayed and asked for a sign that I should be a professional baseball player because of all the wonderful things I could do and the people I could touch. Five minutes later, I blew out my right knee. Later I was playing baseball in college and I prayed the same prayer again. Fifteen seconds later, I was coming into home plate and blew out my left knee. I told Dr. De Wet about these incidents, and he laughed and said, "Your knees signify direction in life." All this time I had been looking for direction, and my body was trying to compensate and answer my questions as best as it could."

Chapter Two:
Your Grandmother Made You Fat: Epigenetics

"The biological brain does not differentiate between actual, symbolic, or imaginary lack."

-Dr. Pieter De Wet

Obesity is not what we think it is. The brain and our cells are influenced by much more than just our life experiences. Our biology is also influenced by our genealogical patterns. We inherit much of our biological programming from previous generations, including our parents, grandparents, and great-grandparents. Most of us have no inkling about how much influence our genealogy impacts our beliefs and our health. For example, if you suddenly find yourself becoming obese at the age of 20 after having a relatively healthy lifestyle, it is possible that genealogical programming might be responsible or at the very least, be a strong contributor. If you look back through your family history, you may discover that something happened to a key ancestor of yours at possibly that same age of 20. For example, if your grandmother lost a baby when she was 20 years old and this represented a massive trauma reverberating through your family tree from that point on, it could contribute to the programming for your shift in weight at age 20.

3 Critical Elements that Program for Obesity

There are three critical elements that come into play in order to program for obesity.

Personal Unresolved Conflicts

First, there are unresolved conflicts that result from the experiences we go through in life that can cause our bodies to become programmed for obesity. This aspect was covered thoroughly in chapter one.

Pre-Development Conflicts

Second, what happened during the time span that encompasses the nine months before our conception, the average of nine months while we were in the womb, and the first 12 months of our lives creates another critical element that needs to be understood. This is the period during which we get programmed with our life project and purpose. It is called the "project purpose." Most people who develop obesity later in life have the critical elements of programming that are taken on during this critical period of time. This occurs because the experiences their mother and father go through because of unresolved and uncommunicated psychological and biological conflicts of their child. This is present in the subconscious of the child or even at the epigenetic level in the cells. In the cell program of that child, he or she will often exhibit indirectly, the unresolved psychological conflicts of the parent. The unresolved conflicts of the parents become the biological conflicts of the child.

Epigenetic Conflicts

The third critical element that needs to be understood and addressed is family history. It is estimated that 95% of congenital diseases are related to epigenetic programming or imprinting and only about 5% are based on abnormal or defective genetic codes. In other words, most congenital diseases occur as a result of epigenetically programmed gene expression and not gene defects. What does epigenetics mean? The definition of epigenetics, simply stated, states that we come into life predisposed to diseases such as obesity. These predispositions are not because we have defective genes or DNA. Rather, they originate from the survival dramas and traumatic experiences that our ancestors suffered. These are the events that literally programmed us for many of the health challenges that we end up dealing with.

Epigenetic programming is not necessarily negative, either. Epigenetic programming is critical for survival because it literally programs us to increase our chances for survival from generation to generation. For example, if starvation occurred in one generation, it's biologically useful for coming generations to be programmed to fatten up more easily when abundance is present in order to decrease the chance of starvation in the case that scarcity occurs. It is critical to understand the relationship between biological and generational wounds. Epigenetics does not care about the individual, but is directed toward survival of the species. It is primarily concerned with the continuation of the genetic pool represented by the family. We are all affected by epigenetic programming from those who have come before us in order to increase the likelihood of survival of future generations.

Your Life Story

There are a number of psychological conflicts, emotional conflicts, and traumatic experiences during one's lifetime that can program for obesity. What's critical to understand is the "felt" experience is relevant and not the lived experience. It is important to remember that no two people are the same in how they experience any event in life that they might go through. Two people can go through the same trauma, and one can program for obesity and the other can program for anorexia. This wide range of results is due to the total difference in the way the subconscious mind deals with the trauma. In other words, the experience might be identical and the manifestations might be exactly the opposite. A good analogy would be when two people go on a roller coaster. While one person might be absolutely horrified, the other experiences exhilaration from going through the very same experience. That is how disease programming works. Before we uncover why that is, let's discuss how it happens.

In the body, a conflict that programs for disease is like a three stage rocket. We mentioned this in chapter one, but let's examine it on a deeper level.

- Stage 1: High stress event.
- Stage 2: The automatic brain manages the conflict (by taking the conflict out of the conscious mind and transferring it into the subconscious mind and into the body)
- Stage 3: Manifestation of the programming as a physical or emotional condition.

Stage One. What happens psychologically, emotionally, and physically? If a woman is attacked and raped, it causes massive emotional stress associated with the direct physical consequences of the attack. This may include possible injury to her thighs and hips as is common with a sexual attack. All three domains (psychological, emotional and physical) are affected.

Stage Two. The automatic brain takes over when the emotion threatens to overwhelm the conscious mind and the brain itself. This automatic brain is responsible for the downloading of the conscious stressor into the subconscious when the trauma or stress threatens to overwhelm consciousness. Failure to run this program could lead to the circuitry in the brain and the nervous system being literally blown out. Much like electrical wiring in a house getting blown out and causing a fire, the same result occurs in an overstressed person. Homes are required to have circuit breakers and so do we.

The brain has its own set of breakers that will activate like a circuit breaker switch in the event of a massive stress-based threat. Our circuit breaker prevents the "fire" of emotional overwhelm to affect the consciousness of the entire brain. The circuit breaker will switch off a particular part of the brain that is related to a specific conflict taking place (the resulting felt experience). There is a connection between a *specific* stress, the specific way we *experience* the stress, the part of the brain that it *links* to, and the specific disease that is *launched* as a result.

In some instances, the conflict is so overwhelming that it is kept in the brain and the brain does not download it, which may cause a nervous breakdown or literally a frying of the wiring inside the brain. The second mechanism, which is far more common, is when the brain downloads to a smaller part of itself and into the body, thereby saving the person's life because it helps them to focus on immediate survival in spite of what has just happened to them. (I.e. In the case of the rape victim, who in spite of the trauma, has to continue on with her life) We can't afford to sit in a corner for the rest of our lives like a blubbering idiot because of what has happened.

Stage Three. The third stage of the conflict occurs when this conflict is downloaded to the body itself and the tissues change as a result. The trauma itself and the way it is experienced in terms of the health experience, literally have the potential to change the expression of the genes within the cell thanks to epigenetic mechanisms. The subconscious program tells the cells, for example, to retain or make fat. Very often it doesn't matter how much or how little a person eats. The fat cells can literally create more fat in line with the conflict that programs for the fattening.

Since family memories can be transferred at the epigenetic level, the traumas and emotional conflicts of your forefathers can echo through the genealogical tree and contribute to the development of obesity in current generations.

Conflicts Programming for Obesity

Our programming for disease comes from three spheres of our existence: the experiences of our own lives starting from the age of one year; the experiences of our parents just before conception, during pregnancy, and up to one year of age; and the experiences of our ancestors, in other words, those who preceded us into the world. When we talk about the conflicts programming for obesity, we do so in the context of one or more of these three aspects.

For instance, a conflict can result from a physically or emotionally traumatic experience that occurs, for example, sometime during childhood or later on. It can be something that happened to our parents while we were in the womb, or it could be a conflict that happened to a family member we are linked with that was not or has not been resolved during their lifetime and that caused an intense conflict for them.

The Conflict of Abandonment

One of the most powerful conflicts programming for obesity is the conflict of abandonment. At the very basic level, abandonment is often related to our relationship with our mother. Biologically, infants and most newborn mammals cannot survive in nature without their mother or a surrogate mother, and therefore are vulnerable to abandonment. In modern human society, that same rule applies. It doesn't matter that we have more safety nets for those coming into this world who do not have a biological mother available. Abandonment can occur if the mother gives birth to a child, gives the baby to a surrogate to raise or pays very little attention to her baby. Even if she keeps the baby, the baby will experience abandonment. When a mother chooses not to breastfeed, it can and almost always does lead to a level of conflict of abandonment. A program of abandonment can be linked to food, for instance, in the case of the mother not breastfeeding the child, or it can be linked to motherly love, for instance, in the case of absence of the mother by choice (i.e. If the mother has someone else holding or feeding the baby for her most of the time). Even if a mother does not abandon her child physically, but in a virtual or symbolic sense, it can program for obesity.

A conflict can be inherited or taken on directly from life's experiences, and it can be related to a reality or be an imaginary, symbolic, or even a virtual experience. A symbolic abandonment may include the failure of the mother to breastfeed or even the failure to breastfeed long enough. If a mother stays home with her baby for three months after they are born, breastfeeding and constantly doting on them, and then suddenly returns to work and ends up switching the baby to formula, the baby will experience a conflict of abandonment, especially if the mother goes back to work by choice. If the mother has to go back to work by necessity and is torn between her baby and work, the biological brain will experience it in a slightly different manner. In this case, it is experienced as a conflict of separation and does not necessarily program for obesity.

The connection between a mother and her baby is made through the skin and is especially powerful when made through the breast. It is natural for a mother to be holding the baby more often when she is breastfeeding the baby than at other times. This may be a very critical reason why babies that have been breastfed long enough have a much lower likelihood of obesity. It is also important to understand that when the mother suddenly disappears for whatever reason, a baby does not have an intellectual understanding as to *why* their mother is not there and therefore will experience either abandonment or separation. When a baby experiences abandonment, biologically, it will enhance its own survival by storing more food as compensation for the abandonment that may result in starvation when exposed to natural environments. That is simply how biology works in nature. In the natural environment, even a momentary lapse of focus on a baby can lead to a loss of the baby to natural enemies.

A conflict of abandonment, of course, happens on a subconscious level because obviously a baby is not able to intellectualize their experiences like an adult might be able to. Essentially, when the baby experiences abandonment, the automatic brain will take this conflict from consciousness and download the experience to a smaller part of the brain and into the body—into the organ that is most resonant with the particular conflict.

Another link in the chain of obesity and the gaining of excess weight has to do with compensatory practices of adults in our society who compensate for their choices. For example, working parents with young children tend to spoil their little ones, oftentimes with food (treats) in order to allay their guilt for time lost with them. When food is used in this way, these so-called "treats" that we feed our kids become linked with this conflict of abandonment in another way, which often programs for addictions that accompany obesity. For example, if our mother feeds us candy in order to allay her guilt, we, in turn, link candy with experiences of abandonment. Every time we go through abandonment later in life, we try to allay that feeling of abandonment with foods that are linked to abandonment in this way. We, quite literally, get programmed for certain foods that become "comfort food." In the subconscious mind, when we feel abandoned in a relationship later on in life, we have a subconscious yearning for mother's love or that which is a substitute for mother's love. Sweet foods like candies are often subconsciously linked to the sweetness of mother's love or the absence of the sweetness of life.

Another way in which this conflict of abandonment plays out is as follows: Biologically, when a baby animal is abandoned by its mother, the baby will do whatever it can to make itself stand out as much as possible in order to make itself noticed. In the animal world when a bear cub is abandoned by its mother, it gets nervous because of that abandonment. It will stand up on its back legs and make itself as tall and visible as possible so that the mother can see it and come back. In the same way, the biological brain will encode for a program of enlargement of the physical body so the abandoned child will be noticed more by its mother and will thereby get its needs for love and affection fulfilled.

When an animal of any kind is abandoned by its mother, it is at much greater risk of dying. Abandoned animals are natural prey for nearly all predators. This creates a clear reason for enlargement programming. The bigger a prey is, the less vulnerable is appears to a potential enemy or predator. This is an additional reason for a bear cub to be able to stand tall when being stalked by a predator such as a mountain lion. It does so in an effort to intimidate the predator into looking for food elsewhere. A blowfish does something similar by blowing itself up as big as possible when it feels threatened, just like the subconscious mind does in a human being who feels threatened, especially if this feeling of threat is linked to abandonment.

Felt Experience Versus Lived Experience

We need to remember that it is the felt experience that is important—not the lived experience. The very same experience in one child may be framed as abandonment and in another child as separation. We mentioned earlier that if the child frames the experience as abandonment, for example, he is more likely to code for obesity. If the child frames it as separation, more likely to code for eczema. Again, this is where the intent of the mother is critical because subconsciously even a baby knows whether the mother wants to be around or not. When the mother does not want to be around the child, it programs for abandonment, but if she can't be with the baby because of circumstances, it programs for separation.

It is critical for a baby at a biological level to be able to distinguish energetically or subconsciously between being abandoned versus a separation occurring. A child who has been abandoned is placed at much more risk than a child who has suffered separation. In the case of abandonment, it usually means that there is an absent-minded parent who does not feel a strong biological bond with their child. In separation, that biological bond tends to be very strong, causing a mother to be more discerning on whom she asks to help take care of her child.

At a biological level the brain of an adult who experiences abandonment at the hands of family will encode that conflict just like the brain of a baby that is abandoned by the mother. For example, a father who works a lot of hours to make ends meet and keep the family afloat financially might be married to a woman and have children who may not show their appreciation to him very regularly, causing him to feel emotionally abandoned. He may end up spending more and more time working and away from his family, and the conflict of abandonment ends up adding weight to his body as a symbolic replacement for the love and appreciation he is lacking. On a biological level, the brain does not necessarily differentiate between a lack of food and a lack of love. Many times the brain substitutes food for love, becoming a major driver for obesity.

Another example of an adult experiencing abandonment programming for obesity would be a woman who goes through an emotionally-charged divorce. She marries a man she believes will take care of her and the babies that she's going to have with him. She ends up being deeply disappointed because of her dependence on him. Her attitude declines and becomes a catalyst for him to seek approval elsewhere. The man goes out drinking with his buddies virtually every night, causing her to feel more and more abandoned by him emotionally and physically. She files for divorce, even though she was the one who felt emotionally abandoned by him. During the initial phase of separation, called the conflict active phase, she may end up losing weight because of the severe stress, causing her to not want to eat. She may show other signs of stress, including insomnia, cold hands and feet, and irritability. After a while, she will eventually get to a relative peace of mind about the separation and divorce and at that moment may start gaining weight in line with the conflict of abandonment that is still present at this level. I explained how these different phases, including the conflict active phase and the healing or recovery phase, all work in my first book, *Heal Thyself: Transform Your Life, Transform Your Health*.

In this example, when her divorce has been finalized and all the lawyers have been paid and she's able to go on with her life, she will tend to move into what is called the healing or recovery phase of the conflict and she will start gaining weight. It is important to understand that fat tissue will literally become *thinner* during the conflict active phase, whereas during the healing or recovery phase, the fat cells will start filling up and dividing. This process to make more fat cells is designed to compensate biologically for the abandonment that has been suffered. Her biology *knows* that she may have to raise her kids now on her own with less support, so she is going to have to store more calories for leaner times in order to be there in strength and stamina for her kids.

Substitutes for Abandonment

We previously discussed how certain foods can link up with a conflict of abandonment. The substitute linked to abandonment is defined by our experiences in life. For example, if our mother tried to allay her guilt of abandoning us by giving us candy, we will link candy to the experience of abandonment. On the other hand, if she stops breastfeeding us too early or never breastfeeds us, we may link abandonment with milk and become dairy addicts. Sometimes we crave substances that will literally alter our moods because of the depression often resulting from abandonment, which may lead to an association between that conflict of abandonment and drugs or alcohol.

Certain items also lead to additional weight gain because of the calories inherent in them. For instance, alcohol has the same number of calories per ounce as fat does, which is about nine calories per ounce. This is why alcohol is more likely to lead to weight gain and obesity, at least in the early phases of addiction to alcohol. We mentioned sweets being a substitute for love earlier, which is why some people turn to chocolate or other sweets. Dairy may be a substitute for motherly love because dairy products are subconsciously linked to mothers. We crave dairy subconsciously when we go through a conflict of abandonment by the mother because dairy is symbolic of mothers. Mom is critical to the survival of the baby through her breast milk, biologically. It's only in recent times that we've had the luxury of not having to breastfeed. Previously if you couldn't breastfeed, the baby died automatically.

If we have enough of a mother but the mother that we have is not well-balanced, we may develop an addiction to processed dairy. Processed dairy includes foods like cheese, yogurt, and ice cream. With cravings for processed dairy, it is not necessarily related to feeling completely abandoned by the mother but rather emotionally or intellectually abandoned by her. Someone may have grown up in their mother's house through their childhood and teenage years, but their mother may not have been emotionally available or mature enough to be there for them emotionally. This causes the person to experience an abandonment that is related to the mother's nature. Addictions to processed forms of dairy are frequently linked to the quality of the relationship between the child and the mother.

We can contrast the addiction to processed dairy with the addiction to normal dairy, which may occur if a mother abandoned her child early on in their life. For example,

- Mother left her marriage and her child behind
- The child was raised in an orphanage
- Mother left the child in daycare every day for the first five years of the child's life even though she didn't need to

In any of these scenarios, that child may develop an addiction for milk itself rather than processed dairy.

Food addictions have a link with the conflict of abandonment but may also be linked to the conflict of separation. For instance, if my father emotionally abandoned me or was not emotionally available to me, and was too tired to interact with his children, it may be experienced as a conflict of separation or abandonment. Either one of these scenarios may program for an addiction to wheat. Wheat is symbolic of the sun, and the sun is symbolic of father. The reason for this is because wheat can only be grown in full sun, which means the field that it grows in has to get sun from dusk to dawn every day. That's why you will never see trees in a wheat field. This also explains why abandonment or separation from father is linked with conditions such as wheat allergies, wheat sensitivities, and diseases like celiac disease or celiac sprue, which can cause intestinal or neurological problems. A conflict of separation from father rather than a conflict of abandonment from father often leads to a double whammy of wheat sensitivity (gluten sensitivity) combined with wheat addiction, which is a very common twist.

Corn and other grains have a lot in common with wheat. Grains are unique in the sense that they are easier to grow for long periods of time to increase the likelihood of long term survival. When we go through survival crises, like when we have too little money, too little love, or too little support, then the subconscious links that experience to grains, leading to cravings for grain-based foods.

If you think about the Israelites crossing the desert from Egypt to what is now called Israel, they had to have grains to sustain them through the desert because there were no fruits or vegetables. There were no crops that they could harvest on their journey. They were dependent on bread and the grains they could make bread from. In the same way, biologically, when we go through scarcity or adversity, we are programmed not only to be drawn to grains, but also to store them. The storing of grains isn't simply in our homes and pantries, but in our bodies as well.

When the body goes through adversity, abandonment, or scarcity, it will attempt to store those calories. This manifests by turning the metabolism down so that we can get through leaner times without burning all of our *resources* and be left with nothing. Biologically, the brain cannot distinguish between a primitive situation and a modern situation. It perceives them in the same way. We are biologically programmed for survival, and that's one reason why humanity has populated the earth to the point that it has. We are incredible survivors, and included in the survival tools is the ability for us to store calories on a whim, literally by flipping a switch whenever scarcity arrives or is perceived. Even if we are living in ostensible abundance with grocery stores on virtually every corner, our primitive mind has not yet adapted to modern abundance.

It is also important to realize that grain addictions are also linked to survival in another way. Grains, especially refined grains, tend to be easily digestible, making it easy for the body to digest and store the calories embedded in these foods. Many people are more likely to be addicted to white bread and processed grains than whole grains because whole grains take a lot more energy to digest and absorb than processed grains do.

Sugar Shock

We mentioned earlier in this chapter that sugar is linked with the need for 'sweetness' in life. If a child was abandoned or separated from its mother, the brain will often crave not just a sweet because of the sweetness in life, but also because of the easy calories it represents. Sugar provides short bursts of energy which are vital in dramas where imminent danger lurks and immediate survival is at stake. The brain will be drawn to those foods that are high in calorie content and very easy to process and absorb. The ultimate easily-processed substance is sugar. We often crave sugar when we need an immediate boost. The threat doesn't have to be an attack by a saber-tooth tiger. Oftentimes, an emotional challenge, as in a relationship, may involve the need for a sugar boost to provide instant fuel for the fight or flight response.

Sugar in not only involved with 'fight or flight' mode. It is also linked to the main conflict behind diseases such as diabetes. The programming conflict of diabetes involves massive *resistance* with a component of *repugnance*. Repugnance means that something *stinks* in my territory, so I have to resist massively. For instance, if someone is in a bad marriage where there is a lot of fighting every day, the brain perceives the need to have lots of sugar available in the bloodstream for that fight.

An adolescent who grows up in a family where everybody is fighting and battling will be in fight mode by definition. His conflict will program him to either hide or disappear. The child will either act as big as possible in order to enter the fight (programs for obesity) or acts as small as possible and try to disappear (programs of anorexia).

The addiction to artificial sweeteners falls under the same category as addiction to sweets because the brain cannot distinguish between real sugar and artificial sweeteners. In fact, the whole idea behind the artificial sweetener industry is to fool the brain to believe you are eating sugar when you are not. Because artificial sweeteners have no calories in them, people start ingesting huge amounts of artificial sweeteners in an effort to get that sugar that the brain is craving. Artificial sweeteners are often more addictive than sugar. It's not unusual to see somebody addicted to artificial sweeteners drinking 10 or 12 artificially sweetened soft drinks a day to fulfill that subconscious biological need. It is also not unusual to see those addicted to artificial sweeteners ingesting other calories from processed grains on top of their artificial sweeteners. This will become more understandable when we talk about hormones and physiological responses to certain substances such as sugar or fake sugars.

The Conflict of Aesthetics

Another conflict that commonly programs for obesity is the conflict of aesthetics, also known as the conflict of the silhouette or the conflict of the mirror. Let's see how this all comes together to contribute to the problem of weight gain.

The conflict of aesthetics resembles a self-fulfilling prophesy. When you get to the point of becoming self-conscious of your body shape or body weight, regardless of what that body shape or that body weight is, there is a level of stress that begins to take hold. It is associated with your interpretation of what you see when you look in the mirror. This conflict is interlinked with our cultural norms and perspectives, which change over time.

Historically speaking, voluptuousness was seen as a sign of beauty and health in earlier societies. In today's society, it's framed as a sign of ugliness and a lack of willpower. Our U.S. culture and most of the cultures of the Western World seem to prefer thinness over voluptuousness, especially among young women, sometimes to the extreme, although there seems to be a shift happening in recent years. We also tend to tie our self-worth, self-esteem, and self-confidence to the number on the scale or the inches around the waist. We allow physical phenomena like love handles or saddlebags, to endlessly torment us. So a vicious cycle occurs, which means that the more weight we gain and the more subcutaneous fat we accumulate, the less self-esteem we have compared to those times when we weighed less and carried less fat.

The conflict of aesthetics is, therefore, a conflict of self-devaluation. We attack ourselves symbolically because of what we see reflected in a mirror, or through other people's eyes. We literally project our own judgment upon others even when there is very little or no evidence that they are judging us. Paradoxically, when we carry a conflict of aesthetics, it is analogous to attacking self and needing to protect ourselves, which translates to adding more fat to our frame. When we begin to fear what other people think of us, we start to feel like they are attacking us, even by a casual glance.

The conflict of aesthetics dovetails with the conflict of abandonment. Because of our self-judgment about our body shape or body weight, we fear abandonment associated with the fear of rejection and the fear of separation.

Studies show us that this is more often a problem for women than it is for men. For example, by the age of 12, 70 percent of girls think they are overweight, even though less than 15 percent of them actually are. More than half of girls age 12 and older have already been on at least one diet. Not only are they seeing themselves as overweight, but they are going on diets when there is absolutely no need. It is this cultural mindset that results in the conflict of aesthetics or the conflict of the mirror, even when we are not actually obese or even at the risk of obesity.

Americans are much more likely to develop a conflict of aesthetics than people in other parts of the world. Africa, Asia, and even Europe don't have the same beliefs Americans do. In fact, in many African countries, it is attractive to be overweight because it is perceived as a sign of health. A man in those cultures would be more sexually attracted to a more voluptuous woman. His subconscious beliefs and cultural norms tell him that she will be healthier through childbirth and pregnancy. Moreover, she will be more likely to bear and raise healthy children. The culture of excessive thinness in America does not make biological sense. Chances of problems occurring with pregnancy and child rearing increase with extreme thinness, just as it does with extreme obesity. In other words, a woman who is near anorexic is probably not going to be successful in having and rearing many children.

For the African-American population, there seems to be a greater tolerance and even a fondness for larger body types and higher body weight. This attraction seems to be biologically meaningful and purposeful because larger buttocks, for example, are associated with bigger hips, which, in turn, means an easier time in childbirth. Bigger breasts (not culturally exclusive) are associated with an easier time with child rearing because of the increased ability to breastfeed. This may also explain why there continues to be a strong demand for breast implants and for buttocks enhancement (or butt lifts).

Fertility, in other words, equals attractiveness in these cultures. In many other countries, however, as in the United

States, that is somewhat distorted because of the excessive focus on thinness.

Despite the obvious obesity increase, there is also mounting research showing that our preconception with weight is overblown. It is now abundantly clear that somebody who is seen as overweight can be and often is as healthy as some at normal or ideal weight in spite of our beliefs that any excess weight is associated with illness. Instead of weight being the issue, the habits and associated risk factors are more likely to be associated with illness. Of course, moderate to severe obesity does correlate with a dramatic increase in associated health challenges.

If you are overweight but eat a very healthy diet—you're not eating partially hydrogenated fats, processed grains or artificial sweeteners—you have just as much of a likelihood to be healthy as a thinner person who is eating the same way. As a matter of fact, a thinner person eating junk is far more likely to be unhealthy than a more overweight person eating very healthy. Emotions have a huge impact on this, and we need to realize that obesity is tied to certain emotional conflicts, but so are other diseases that are often linked to obesity. Even though there is congruence between programming for conditions like diabetes, hypertension, hyperlipidemia, and obesity, there are also differences. Somebody who is obese may not have these other conflicts programming for other diseases and may be in exceptionally good health. Whereas somebody else who is minimally overweight may be in seriously poor health because of their disease programming related to their other conflicts and their tendencies toward more dysfunctional lifestyles and greater toxicity levels.

In America, there is a notable aesthetic disconnect between men and women. Millions of women see themselves as unattractive even though they are seen in a very different light by the men in their worlds. Unfortunately, this leads to dysfunctional behaviors among females that are disease-promoting instead of health-promoting and that can also be impoverishing. Many women try to buy their way to feeling good through excessive focus on the latest fashions, toxic cosmetics, toxic and expensive hair-dos, and very expensive cosmetic surgery. We have a population of American women who see themselves as unattractive in total contrast to how they are seen by the men in their lives.

It is creating relationship tragedies.

We have to remember that sexy is in the mind of the beholder. It is your choice whether to see yourself as beautiful or ugly, no matter what has happened to your body. You can be 600 pounds and see yourself as beautiful if you develop that frame of mind or you can be an anorexic 80-pounder who is horribly underweight and see yourself as fat and ugly. The key to healing this conflict of aesthetics is to see the 'sexy' and the beauty in you, no matter what your circumstances. Regardless of your weight, relationship history, or romantic successes or failures, your perception creates your beliefs.

Whose Opinion Do You Listen to?

We will talk later in the book about how to change your thoughts, but it takes a spiritual mindset to heal this conflict, which is something that the ego can never do. The ego is virtually incapable of seeing itself as beautiful. Most people don't feel beautiful because of the devaluation they suffer from. This relates to childhood traumas and the genealogical programming that they came into this world with. The greater our understanding of our biology from a Recall Healing perspective, the easier it is for us to take a spiritual perspective on our body weight and shape. Taking a spiritual perspective is also helpful because we are reminded that we were created in God's image and likeness. From this perspective, how is it possible not to see ourselves as beautiful, attractive, and sexy? On the other hand, when we look at ourselves through the eyes of our ego, we cannot possibly see the extent of our own beauty or attractiveness. Be mindful of whose opinion you listen to when it comes to the perception of attractiveness.

In my other book, *Heal Thyself: Transform Your Life, Transform Your Health*, I have a number of chapters that explore the realm of emotions, the mental sphere, and the spiritual aspects of healing. I also share the aspects of gratitude, living a purpose-driven life, overcoming loss, and maintaining a sense of humor. Those are the skills and the tools we need to help us frame ourselves as sexy no matter what.

The Conflict of the Indigestible Lack

The third conflict that commonly programs for increased body weight is the conflict of the indigestible lack, which basically means that we *don't* have something we *want* or we *have* something we that we *don't* want (i.e. we want something else). This is often interlinked with a conflict of abandonment or a conflict of separation stemming from early childhood. Two examples would be: if a mother has been breastfeeding her baby but when he is three months of age, she has to go back to work to help support the family (conflict of separation) or another mother decides when her baby is three months old that she just doesn't feel like breastfeeding anymore because it's inconvenient (conflict of abandonment). A couple of other examples of conflict of separation are a mother who abandons her breastfeeding attempts because of the baby's trouble with their sucking reflex or if the baby is premature and being kept in an incubator. In both instances, there ends up being a forced separation between mother and baby to some degree. Breastfeeding creates a vital link between mother and baby and when a mother is unable or unwilling to breastfeed, this very often leads to a conflict of either separation or abandonment, depending on the mother's intent.

In any one of those situations above, the baby will experience a conflict of the indigestible lack because of its inability to access mother's milk, which is the ideal food for a baby. Breast milk is constituted in such a way that it perfectly matches the needs of the infant's body. It has exactly the right amount of protein, the right protein constituents, the right balance of amino acids, the right number of minerals, sugar calories, and so forth. It is constituted to be easily digested by the infant's digestive tract and has critical factors in it that ensure or increase the likelihood of a healthy immune system, healthy bones, and healthy development of the brain and other organs. When there is a failure to provide breast milk for the baby for whatever reason, the infant experiences a clearly, biologically perceptible lack that we call the conflict of the indigestible lack.

A baby who is taken off the breast too early will, for the rest of time, have a subconscious or biological yearning for that perfect food that it never received or that was prematurely removed. The biological program of the infant makes him want breast milk, and his body knows that this is the ideal food for him, so when he is deprived of this and it is replaced with other forms of nutrition like baby formula, then the baby becomes fixated on that food or other foods that are substituted for breast milk. Often times parents will make the mistake of replacing the breast milk, not just with formula, (which is artificial in many ways and has added sugar and is sweeter than mother's milk) but will also start substituting with other fast foods and processed foods that become linked emotionally in the baby's mind. This compounds the conflict of deprivation that he suffers because of the removal of the breast milk. For instance, if the mother feeds that baby French fries with ketchup, he will be subconsciously fixated on French fries and ketchup throughout the rest of his life. You can probably think of a hundred of other examples of foods that people are fixated on for this reason.

Many of the food addictions we suffer from and that we seem to have no control over stem from those early childhood experiences related to being deprived of mother's milk and the substitution with other foods that get linked with the biological mind. Later in life, whenever that person goes through a conflict of separation or abandonment, that can lead to a craving for these foods. These current experiences are linked in the subconscious mind with earlier experiences of separation or abandonment. It is also interesting to note that a conflict of separation or abandonment can also cause a slowdown of metabolism. In nature, when the existence of an animal is threatened by abandonment or separation, the natural tendency of its metabolism is to slow down in order to conserve calories for the fight for survival that might ensue. The same applies to adults later in life. This is one of the primary reasons people often act like they are starving and will inhale food even though they are surrounded by abundance.

Another example of the conflict of indigestible lack is when somebody deeply craves a relationship, love, attention, or affection, and she cannot obtain it. She will start craving the foods that are symbolic for the love and attention that she did not receive and that were replacements during the abandonment suffered in childhood.

The conflict of the indigestible lack can be real, symbolic, virtual, or imaginary. Often the brain cannot perceive the difference between a dream and reality, so if you are in your bed sleeping and dreaming that you are on a real roller coaster, you experience the same physiological, brain chemistry, and blood flow pattern changes in the brain, just as if you were on the roller coaster in real life. The same applies to symbolic and virtual triggers.

Up to now we've discussed not having something that we want, but of course there is the second possibility of having something we don't want. For example, when someone is married to someone else who is not giving them the affection they desire, but instead abusing them physically or emotionally, a conflict of the indigestible lack can result. It means that they don't want what they have (they want something else), so their bodies expand to symbolically push away that which is not wanted, i.e., the unloving spouse. Or it may expand in an effort to protect against that which is not wanted or desired (conflict of fat—see below).

Often we become fixated on the particular food that replaces whatever we can't get. At first it's a shock to the system when we are forced to consume something that was not desired on a biological level. For instance, for a baby, the body is literally traumatized by providing inappropriate foods to the body when the body is not ready for that food. If you take a two-month old whose body is built to consume breast milk and force that infant to consume foods that are too heavy and too hard for that little digestive tract to digest, it can program for a conflict of the indigestible lack. However, the food that replaces the more ideal food fills a void that exists and becomes linked in the mind to the abandonment or separation that is being suffered at the time.

Emotionally, as stated earlier, whatever food is used to replace that which we can no longer obtain, like mother's breast milk, will cause a fixation. For example, when a duckling hatches from an egg it becomes fixated on the first moving object that it perceives once it leaves the egg. If that object is a human or a robot moving around, it will become fixated on that as if it is his mother in the same way the brain becomes fixated on the food that replaced the breast milk prematurely.

This is often how food addictions develop. If a child, for instance, wants breast milk but is fed something else, the result is often an addiction to that same food later in life. If you want to find the source of that addiction, we have to go back into their childhood and learn about the history of what they were fed as infants and young children. Look at the history of whether or not they were breastfed, if breastfed, when the mother ceased breastfeeding. Examine whether or not any abandonment or separation conflicts were present and what foods might have been used to fill a void during emotional traumas suffered. We also need to find out whether the mother and/or father spent adequate time with the infant and if not, who the surrogate caregiver was. If any form of food was used as a reward or to fill a void during emotional trauma it will have an imprint. This explains many of the most severe food addictions we see in our society and is one of the reasons it is so difficult to overcome bad eating habits and food addictions.

The liver is often the target organ for the conflicts of indigestible lack because biologically the liver is linked with conflicts of scarcity. For example, when a baby is taken off the mother's breast and adequate nutrition for the child's biology is not supplied through other means, the liver often works overtime to store what is ingested. For instance, breast milk contains certain components that are critical for health. If our biology perceives a lack of those components, it will try to find them elsewhere in the foods that are available to us. If we consume sugars from sources other than mother's milk, the liver will try to store that as a counter to the deprivation. If it's fat that is perceived as lacking, it will look for fat in the diet and store or make the fat. In the case of sugar, the liver turns sugar from its original form into what's called glucagon, which is the form sugar is stored in the liver and muscles. The liver will also turn sugar into fat under certain circumstances.

The Conflict of Fat

The fourth conflict that programs for being overweight is the conflict of fat, which basically means that the body uses fat to protect itself for various reasons. This biological brain programs causes the body to create fat in order to become bigger so that it can protect itself and others.

For example, if a woman feels threatened by a man (for example, her husband) because he threatens physical violence upon her when they fight, she may gain weight as a counter to his aggression to protect herself from him.

However, the child of that couple may also experience the same conflict as the mother. The mother's feelings of being threatened by the father will cause the child to gain weight because her biological program is to become a wedge between her father and mother. She does this to protect her mother from her father. Initially this is symbolic because it may take years for her to become big enough in reality to be a wedge or a protector. If she sees threatening behavior from her father, she forms a layer of protection to protect herself as well because of her own fear of violence being directed towards her and not just her mother. This would especially be true if the father acts abusively toward the child. Another example would be if someone is kicked in the stomach by a horse, he may develop a layer of fat right around the area that was injured. In this instance, the body will add fat in that particular area or in the general area. This is the brain's way of programming for protection for the future based on past experiences and will constantly reprogram to adjust to perceived threats from the outer world.

Conflict of Fat as a Hedge Against Starvation

The conflict of fat also comes into play in cases of starvation or threatened starvation in the person or in their genealogy. If you have suffered near starvation at any point during your lifetime, you will take on a conflict of fat. This creates a tendency to store more fat in times of abundance in order to hedge against possible future starvation. For example, if a child develops dysentery at nine months old and almost dies as a result, suffering dramatic weight loss in the process, in later years when a stressful situation occurs, a conflict of fat might kick in based on this original programming conflict of near starvation. The same child who almost died of dysentery, when faced with severe lack at a later age (for example, when going through a divorce from his spouse and suffering severe financial loss as a result), the biology might respond by adding fat as a result of this triggering conflict, which is linked with the programming conflict stemming from the event at nine months old.

Another example would be if the mother experienced near starvation while the child was in her womb because she couldn't find food for a significant period of time. Often, the child will take on the conflict of fat, which means that the child's biological brain acts as a counter to the mother's actual experience of deprivation and starvation. Again, we say that the psychological conflict of the parent becomes the biological conflict of the child, especially those traumas that are not fully processed psychologically by the parents. It is also important to note that if there is a history of a drama leading to starvation in the family, (especially if someone died of starvation) then there will be an epigenetic program for increasing body weight in future generations.

The reason for this programming for increased body weight is to decrease the chances of starvation occurring in future generations. Our genes literally retain epigenetic imprints of the starvation dramas that happened in the past in the family, so the body will store fat as a counter measure. More calories are stored as fat than in any other form in the human body.

Conflict of Fat as a Hedge against Drowning

When there is a history of a near drowning experience or a family history of drowning, the body will protect itself from drowning by triggering more fat storage. The reason for this is because fat is literally a built-in flotation device. Fat is lighter than water and therefore floats on water. Muscle and bone, on the other hand, are heavier than water and tend to sink. Someone who is very lean exerts more energy to stay afloat than someone who is overweight. An example of a trauma leading to central obesity would be a child who suffers a near drowning as a result of slipping out of an inner tube that is too big for him, ending up in the bottom of a pool, and being rescued at the last moment. In later years that same child might grow up with his own built-in inner tube (central obesity), which represents the biological response to falling through the hole in the inner tube, leading to a near-death experience. In this example, when someone falls through a floatation device in the water and nearly drowns, the subconscious mind solves the issue. It prevents it from ever happening again by fattening the body. This conflict is especially important to me, because it is part of my personal experience. At five years old, I nearly drowned.

In 1965, my parents were at a party with a group of people. They had a swimming pool, and I was in the pool with my siblings and some other children. It was a relatively small pool, and there were about 12 children in the pool with me. I was in an inner tube that was too big for me, and while everyone was having a good time, I slipped through the inner tube and ended up on the bottom of the pool where I almost drowned. Thankfully my father looked over the swimming pool fence just in time to see me struggling at the bottom of the pool. I was rescued and resuscitated, but it left an indelible imprint on my subconscious. I had been very thin as a child and still was at age four. When I turned 25 (exactly five times the age when this event occurred), I started gaining significant weight. This started after another near death experience when I was involved in a head-on collision. When I reached 10 times that age (age 50), I went through severe financial turmoil and my weight took off again. These timelines represent mathematical cycles linked to the age at which the near drowning occurred and are correlated with the subsequent increases in my body weight. It was as if my biology was reacting to survival dramas at those previous points in time.

These mathematical cycles and other scientific explanations of how all of this works are described further in my other book *Heal Thyself: Transform Your Life, Transform Your Health.* It explains in great detail how we are programmed for different diseases and how the timing of experiences in our lives have huge importance of what gets programmed, how and when it plays out. Mathematical cycles are very critical in our experience of being human and in our pathologies. For instance, if a woman loses a baby at age 20 and that baby dies at birth, she would obviously be deeply and profoundly traumatized by that. After she gives birth, she will often retain the body weight representing the baby who died. For instance, if the baby weighed 10 pounds at birth, she will find it nearly impossible to lose the final 10 pounds, which represent that traumatic loss. At age 40, double the age of the loss, she may gain another 10 pounds as a result.

The Conflict of Burden

The fifth conflict that commonly programs for increased body weight can be called the conflict of burden, which relates to all of those things in life that we tend to carry and that we feel burdened by. Again, this can be real, imaginary, virtual, or symbolic. An example of this would be a husband and father who develops obesity because of a conflict he experiences in having to take care of his family and/or his business under trying conditions and feels extremely burdened as a result. He tries his best to provide for his family, but somehow he may feel inadequate in that role. For instance, he may not feel that enough appreciation is being shown by his family, or he may perceive employees are unappreciative and may even feel rightly or wrongly that they are stealing from him or abusing his kindness. This all becomes a conflict of burden.

An individual in this kind of situation often feels that there is a gap between what he is giving and what he is getting back. For example, he may feel unacknowledged or unappreciated in contrast to his self-perceived Herculean efforts. If he feels progressively more and more loaded down with the weight of responsibility he carries, this programs for increasing body weight, especially around the midsection of the body (central obesity). Some people call this a 'Buddha complex' because if you look at images of the Buddha, he was depicted as morbidly obese with the weight carried around his middle. That obesity of the Buddha symbolizes the burden that he carried in relation to the suffering of humanity. This is similar to the conflicts that are often carried by mothers, healers, and anyone who has a tendency to take on the emotional burdens of others in any significant way. In this particular situation, obesity is the body's attempt to gain more energy and to have a greater supply of energy available in order to continue carrying the perceived burden. It also symbolizes protection of the solar plexus, which is where we feel emotional vulnerability at the gut level. It is almost like the obesity cushions and protects the solar plexus against emotional insults from those around us who seem unaware of the burdens that we carry on their behalf.

How to Release the Past to Create a New Future

When we look at the conflicts listed and the fact that so many people are afflicted by these types of conflicts, it's no wonder that obesity is becoming more and more of a problem in certain parts of the world. In other words, our stress levels are not decreasing, but increasing as our society becomes more and more complex. Economic, social and family stressors are everywhere. With divorce and separation becoming more and more commonplace, the compounding and reverberating conflicts add up. Not only are we dealing with the conflicts that relate to our personal lives and the content of our lives, but also those that relate to what happened to our parents, our ancestors and our children. In order to overcome and resolve these conflicts and the impact that these conflicts have on us, we must release them in order to create a healthier and more empowering future for ourselves. This is where the science of Recall Healing comes in.

We will talk a great deal more about Recall Healing later in the book, but basically the thought behind Recall Healing is that in order to heal we have to become aware of our life's story. All illnesses and pathologies start with a conflict that threatens to overwhelm the psyche and then is downloaded as a biological program. A biological conflict is, in other words, an unresolved psychological conflict that threatens to overwhelm the conscious mind and is then downloaded to a smaller part of the brain and sometimes, but not always, into the body itself. If it stays in the brain, it becomes a psychiatric health challenge, such as depression, anxiety, or schizophrenia. Or if it downloads to the body, it becomes a physical disease like obesity or diabetes. In order to heal a disease, by definition, we have to deal with it at the root level instead of just dealing with it at the symptom level. That means we have to help the person who is afflicted with the health challenge to become aware of the conflict that is programming for the disease.

Once we are able to name and recall the conflict, we can dump it, which then gives us a much better chance of permanently healing our bodies. By understanding, gaining insight, and releasing our past, we gain the ability to gain a brighter future.

Disease is similar to an iceberg. What you see above the surface is only a visible fraction of your reality. In relative terms, both are illusions. The ocean obscures part of the iceberg underneath the surface just like a disease obscures the deeper roots that are present below the surface. Yet, most people beyond and their physicians are not aware of this.

In order to heal an illness, it is critical and imperative that we discover and resolve the condition at its roots. The roots can be described by looking at the five levels of healing, which include:

- Level One: The Physical Body
- Level Two: The Energy Body
- Level Three: The Mental Body
- Level Four: The Intuitive Body

- Level Five: The Spirit Body

Most healthcare practitioners only focus on Level One, the physical body, but most diseases are sourced at one of the deeper levels. The physical level is where treatments like pharmaceutical interventions, surgery, physical therapy, chiropractic, nutrition, diet, supplements, vitamins, minerals, herbs, and aroma therapy are applied. From a diagnostic perspective, the physical exam, blood work, and genetic testing are all focused on evaluation at this physical level, which is also the level at which certain detoxification strategies are employed to assist the organs of detoxification, including the liver, the kidneys, the lymphatics, and the intestinal tract. We're not negating level one treatment strategies. In fact, it is critical to support the physical vehicle in order to gain enough physical and emotional energy to do higher level work.

Level Two, the energy body relates to physics and physiology. The physical body is surrounded with and penetrated by an energy field, which consists of electromagnetic and gravitational forces, in addition to weak and strong nuclear forces. Electromagnetic devices and light therapies are used to impact on this level. Level two is that part of our being that is also affected most by certain modern technologies, which can contribute to the development of health challenges. For instance, certain types of radiation coming from the electronic devices that we work with on a daily basis can literally make us sick at this level. This is called electromagnetic fog or electromagnetic pollution. Level two, by the way, is also the level involved with many diagnostics performed in conventional medicine. For instance, magnetic resonance imaging (MRI), electrocardiography (EKG), and x-rays are level two strategies that we use to diagnose with every day in conventional medicine. There is a dearth of treatment strategies at this level. The exceptions would be radiation therapy for cancer, the TENS electric unit for pain control, which is an electrical device that literally suppresses pain stimuli, and lasers, which are used more and more in aesthetics to do non-surgical face lifts and help people lose inches, for example.

In natural medicine there are dozens of level two therapies in use, including acupuncture, neural therapy (which involves local anesthetics into local nerve control centers), certain types of homeopathics, and Reiki massage (which has to do with energy field manipulation and balancing). Meditation and yoga are also modalities that play out at this level. (Yoga is both a physical and an energetic modality).

Level Three is what we call the mental body, which is linked to our thoughts, feelings, belief systems, and our perceptions. It is at the mental body where our emotions are organized. This is where unresolved psychological conflicts have their greatest influence. These unresolved conflicts stem from traumatic events that we have experienced in our lives. They form a large part of the root cause of the illnesses we experience. Recall Healing is one of the best evaluation tools used at this level, in which we gather information on past traumatic events which have influenced the body in ways that can promote disease formation.

Other modalities that are used at this level include the analysis of one's belief systems through the use of psychoanalysis, and the use of psycho-kinesiology to evaluate for deep-seated emotions (psycho-kinesiology is a form of muscle testing that helps us to explore the emotional realm, literally by using the muscles of the physical body and responses of those muscles to different inputs, including emotional inputs). Certain aspects of homeopathy or homeopathic healing methods also belong to this level of healing, especially when we talk about what are called flower remedies or high-dilutional remedies (high dilutions of substances). High dilutional remedies and flower remedies impact us at the emotional level.

Level Four is also called the intuitive body and is related to what is called the collective or mass consciousness. This is where epigenetics comes into play. We carry around not only our own unresolved conflicts, but the unresolved conflicts of our ancestors (genealogical wounds), our culture, our race, and even our religions. Generational conflicts can contribute to the development of obesity and are related to what happened to our ancestors going back as many as four generations, including our generation. These genealogical conflicts or epigenetic wounds associated with the development of obesity would include conflicts related to devaluation, separation, threat of attack, or a threat to survival. For example, the loss of love, a loss of respect, or a loss of intimacy that an ancestor experiences could program for disease in coming generations. The threat to survival that our ancestors went through can program for this disease. These influences should be discovered, if at all possible. Knowing about them is the key to resolving the conflicts that program for disease and thereby healing our bodies from disease, including obesity.

Certain healing modalities, including Recall Healing, total biology, Germanic new medicine, and Evox voice analysis are tools that are beneficial in treating level three wounds and issues. All of them, except for Germanic new medicine, are effective for treating level four. When dealing with the intuitive body, the most important thing to focus on is reestablishing love and respect within the family where it has been lost. We can accomplish this best by going back at least four generations, including our own, to resolve any conflicts that program for disease within the family. Any toxic secrets or generational curses within the family should be exposed at this level. Often when we heal something at level four, instant healing at level three may also occur, literally clearing all of the conflicts experienced in our lives stemming from that original genealogical conflict, thereby making it far easier for the body to heal, for example, from issues such as obesity.

As far as the intuitive body is concerned, the good news is that even for those who have no idea what curses lie within the family, healing is possible at this level. This is because of the phenomenon called intuition. Even if you don't know the details of your ancestral stories, you will be able to access some of those generational memories by intuiting what might have happened in the family based on what you are inflicted with health-wise and what has happened to you during your life.

Oftentimes when people start doing this level of discovery, they will have dreams and revelations that help them to get a feeling for what might be hidden in their genealogy. For example, if someone develops obesity at a very young age and is born with hypothyroidism, just knowing what those diseases are normally associated with can help us intuit what might have happened in the womb or in the genealogy. Even in the case of adoption, there may be clues as to what is carried genealogically and through the project purpose. For instance, if an adopted child is born with obesity and a low thyroid, we can intuit the possibility that a huge drama played out while the child was in the mother's womb. Examples may include abandonment by the father of the baby early on in pregnancy, leading to the mother experience abandonment and the baby experiencing abandonment by extension.

Much of the work needed for healing at level three and level four can be done by the individual without help, but it does make a tremendous difference to have someone knowledgeable by your side to help you gain insight and to help your intuition because, as they say, two heads are better than one. Another person can literally evaluate you through psycho-kinesiology to literally bolster your intuition and your ability to tap into the subconscious. You can test someone kinesiologically for the factors related to what happened in the womb and what happened in the genealogy that might be contributing to their disease process.

To learn more about Recall Healing, get a copy of my book *Heal Thyself: Transform Your Life, Transform Your Health.* This is also a series of DVDs available on Recall Healing, including on Levels One, Two, and Three, and a number of disease-specific DVDs for those interested in a more in-depth study of Recall Healing.

Level Five is also called the spirit body, which includes religion, spirituality, and self-help. You have to be able to overcome spiritual challenges in order to be able to heal. This involves nurturing a connection with our higher self, our divine essence, our creator or God. Regardless of how we label this energetic force, we know it is present at the core of our being. Spirit body is linked with the experience of unconditional love, joy, inner peace within ourselves, toward others, and life itself. Level Five healing also has to do with the purification and illumination of our connection with our creator.

At Level Five, healing becomes virtually automatic and can occur spontaneously without even having to try. However, paradoxically, level five healing is also associated with a deeper understanding that we are not our bodies, that the body is just a vehicle and just a tool at our disposal. Therefore it loses its inherent importance. It is also paradoxical that when we work at these higher levels that we lose the fear of death and suffering that is so inherent to the ego.

In order to heal at Level Five, we have to be able to move past our egos and let go of judgment and righteousness. One of the most effective tools that help to bring about healing at Level Five is the attitude of gratitude. Being grateful for everything, including even health challenges such as obesity or illness, truly can make an astronomical difference in what happens to us as far as healing. Prayer, affirmation, and meditation are also very beneficial tools to use at this level.

What's important to understand is that level five healing cannot be taught or given. Level five healing can only be inspired. You show people the way by how you live your life and how you handle adversity. But you should be careful of someone who claims to be able to teach you level five healing or who tries to 'sell' you level five healing strategies. Level five is the level of true self-healing, which means that you have to create a path to communicate with and commune with your higher self, your essence, or your divinity, and no one can do that for you. This is truly the level of profoundly deep self-exploration. To use the tools I have discussed, you literally have to take time away from the stress of life to connect with your creator. That's why meditation is so powerful. Meditation, by definition, takes you out of the business of every day survival. It puts you in a mindset where you are able to quiet the conscious mind and enter the subconscious. This is also the level where it is far more possible to heal the wounds that program for afflictions than when you are so busy and preoccupied with your life, you run around like a scolded twit.

The same applies to prayer. Numerous studies on prayer have shown prayer's benefits in healing. Research has repeatedly shown that praying for others helps them to heal. Interestingly, it has also concluded that it also helps those who are doing the praying for others. When you pray for someone else's healing with no thought to your own healing, you will paradoxically find yourself healed from your afflictions, as well as those you prayed for. There was a study done on AIDS patients in San Francisco, in which groups of people from different religions and different denominations were put together to pray for specific patients with AIDS. Prayers were done for enhancement of certain parameters, for instance, to increase white cell count or to increase CD 4 counts, or to reduce biological markers of inflammation of the body. They also looked at overall happiness and other health parameters in the study. They studied not only the health of those who were being prayed for, but also those who were doing the praying and found extraordinary, truly fascinating findings. Notably, those who were doing the praying actually were responding *even more* than those who were being prayed for, and the response occurred in more categories than in those who were being prayed for.

Both prayer and meditation take you more into an alpha brain wave activity pattern rather than beta wave brain activity pattern. A preacher once noted that prayer and meditation are two sides of the same coin: "Prayer is when you talk to God; meditation is when you listen to God."

In summary it is important for us to realize that in order to heal obesity, we must discover and clear the disease at its roots. This means that we have to access its source at level three, four or five in order to be able to heal long-term. When you work at a higher level than the original insult, you may paradoxically be able to heal much more readily than at the level at which the insult occurred. For instance, even though something might have originated at Level Three, by doing work at Levels Four and Five, you may facilitate the healing dramatically. This is a way to exponentially increase the power of healing. This concept also applies to the investment it takes to heal. If all you do are Level One healing strategies, the cost will be prohibitive and the success will be shallow and temporary, at best. You will keep expending fortunes as you cycle back and forth, losing and gaining weight repeatedly, getting sicker and sicker in the process. If you invest in Level Two strategies, your expenditures will tend to go down, traction will be gained and more progress will be made. However, it is not until you really start investing in and applying yourself to Level Four and Level Five strategies that long-term healing becomes much more likely and endless cycles of failure become much less likely.

Veronica Smith (name has been changed) has as of this printing lost over 145 pounds and reversed hypothyroidism, lower back pain, degenerative disc disease, joint problems, high blood pressure, and severe obesity of the thighs, knees, buttocks, upper back, upper arms, chin, etc. She has also overcome a large amount of emotional baggage to achieve what she has.

###

Sometimes when you are facing multiple health challenges, it's hard to know where to begin. Several years back I went through two physically abusive relationships. I suffered a separated shoulder, back and neck injuries, a broken nose and a concussion just to name a few. I had also been raped, stabbed, and left for dead earlier in my life at one point. Needless to say, my physical body is not all that went through the traumas. My mind, emotions, will, and spirit was equally impacted by these events.

Little did I know that not only had these events imprinted on my metabolism, physical and emotional health, but factors in the lives of my mother and grandmother had also drafted a blueprint of how I was to lead and live my life.

As the years passed, my body continued to slowly break down, and then my husband's health began failing and I also started down the path as caregiver for my aging parents while still trying to maintain a full time job. I became so acclimated to being in pain, no energy, overweight, low metabolism, that I attributed these symptoms to being tired and stressed. My attention was focused on everyone else. My mentality was their health challenges were worse than what I was going through that I did not hear what my body was trying to tell me. My body spoke loud and clear one day when my adrenal system completely crashed on me. It threw me into a seizure-like episode and total collapse of energy and strength to took hours to pass.

This was my wake-up call.

As I began working with Dr. De Wet and we did a wide array of testing—both conventional as well as bio-energetic testing. My results were a wake-up call, and in a way, a road map. This is where I am, so I know where my starting point is and where I am wanting to go. I weighed 305 pounds, my adrenal system was shot, my thyroid was almost non-functional even though I was on the largest dose of Armour Thyroid that can be prescribed, and my hormones were all off balance. I learned that one of those hormones deficiencies alone could impact many systems, let alone a whole bunch of them. The coup de gras was my cardiac results. I knew someone who was 13 years older than me and who had been through open heart surgery twice, and my cardiac workup results were worse than that person.

How did I get to this point?

Finding the answers to that question and resolving it is a large part of the story to follow. Dr. De Wet employed numerous treatment strategies in the care that he provided to help me get these health challenges under control. Some of them included the β HCG Weight Loss Program, nutritional guidelines, Segment Therapy (which combines acupuncture, Mesotherapy, neural therapy, and a technique called "nappage" with injectable local anesthetics, injectable homeopathics, and injectable nutrients, including vitamin B12). We targeted my adrenal glands, my thyroid, and numerous other organ systems. We also used the same treatment to reset my shoulders, neck and back. Coupled with supplements and a bio-identical hormone prescription, I began to improve.

These previous steps started me on my way to recovery. As I began this path of recovery, I made a commitment to myself that I would not let anything stand in the way of my healing—including myself. I knew this healing journey would not be easy. I was facing major challenges: physically, mentally, and emotionally. The beauty of true, in-depth, holistic healing is getting down to the root cause of health challenges and treating it at that level. I had reached the point in my life that I didn't want to just treat symptoms and feel better for a while; I wanted complete healing on all levels.

As I continued working with Dr. De Wet, we took a hard

look at the events of my life, my conflicts about those events, and how those conflicts literally opened the door for the health challenges I have been facing. This is called Recall Healing, and I can only tell you that it has allowed me to heal in ways I only dreamed of—in-depth, to the core healing, getting down to the cause, and either reframing or resolving my conflicts. This is complete freedom for the mind and emotions that, in turn, creates the healing opportunity for the body!

By approaching my healing on all five levels, I now have these results to celebrate and shout about: my emotional and mental healing, which set the stage for the following results: I lost 145 pounds, my thyroid gland and adrenals are all working optimally (without prescription medications), and my metabolism has been restored. My degenerative disc disease has resolved, my joints are all better, and my blood pressure is resolved.

Please note that I listed the mental and emotional healing most prominently since I am convinced it formed the most critical part of my overall healing. Don't settle for partial healing: reach for the OPTIMAL and ULTIMATE HEALING. Allow yourself to enter this space, embrace it, and drive right through to the healthiest you. This kind of healing is attainable and worth every step you make and every change you incorporate.

Chapter Three:
Turning Your Metabolism into a Nuclear Reactor

"We can turn our bodies into massive calorie-burning furnaces by simply changing our beliefs about what is good for us and acting on those beliefs."

-Dr. Pieter De Wet

When you want to turn the body you have into the body you want, it is critical to learn how to optimize calorie burning and turn your metabolism into a calorie-burning furnace. In order to accomplish this, we must look into repairing dysfunctional beliefs, clearing negative processing, and resolving negative emotions. All of these tend to slow down our metabolism. In this chapter, we will be revealing key steps towards accomplishing this mission. First on the agenda is to learn how to process emotions properly. A lot of people think that positive thinking represents the main emotional tool towards better health and losing weight, but that is over simplistic and largely untrue. You can't simply be a positive thinker and disregard or negate your negative emotions and the negative thoughts associated with them. Our emotions are tied directly to our thoughts and beliefs, so these negative thoughts have to be processed and worked through before they can be resolved. Just shoving them aside does not allow us to actually deal with them. The beliefs are still there, along with the manifestations they create. Conscious positive thinking has almost zero effect on your beliefs or illness. We must examine our thoughts and beliefs at a deeper level in order to change or redirect them.

The Impact of Emotions on Metabolism

There is a relative connection between the slowing of metabolism and negative emotions and between the speeding up of metabolism and positive emotions. Theoretically we can turn our bodies into massive calorie-burning furnaces by simply changing what we believe. Our beliefs are the drivers of our emotions, feelings, and interpretations of the universe that we live in. The object in reforming or healing a broken metabolism is to learn to generate more positive emotions more *consistently*. It is inherently very difficult to accomplish this when we have engrained counterproductive belief systems that correlate with the creation of negative emotions.

Generating positive emotion is critical for healing. In Dr. David Hawkins' book *Power Versus Force*, he lays out a map of consciousness, which shows how every emotion is associated with a certain level of energy. Negative emotions are low energy emotions, and positive emotions correlate with higher energy. For instance, one loving thought is ten thousand times more powerful than one guilty thought. One peaceful thought is ten thousand times more powerful than one fearful thought.

Think of it as a ladder with each rung on the ladder representing certain energy levels which correlate with certain thoughts, beliefs, feelings, perspectives on how we look at the world, and even how we perceive our creator to be. The bottom rung of the ladder would correlate with the lowest energy emotions, represented by the most negative emotions with the most negative impact on our health. As we climb from the bottom rung to the higher rungs on this ladder, we become better able to heal from diseases, whether they are physical, emotional, or mental. We also become much better at healing our metabolisms, among other things, as we climb this ladder toward more and more empowering emotions. The more empowering emotions we generate, the more likely we are to have healthier metabolisms and to be healthier overall. Here in ascending order are the 17 levels as represented on Dr. Hawkins' map of consciousness, with level one representing the lowest energy and level 17 representing the highest energy:

1. Shame
2. Guilt
3. Apathy
4. Grief
5. Fear

6. Desire

7. Anger

8. Pride

9. Courage

10. Neutrality

11. Willingness

12. Acceptance

13. Reason

14. Love

15. Joy

16. Peace

17. Enlightenment

Attached to the levels on the map of consciousness are specific emotions and typical actions. For instance, at the level of shame, humiliation is the most common emotion, and self-destruction and destruction toward others would be common actions. The next level is guilt, with blame associated with it. The following correlations are also readily apparent:

Apathy = despair; grief = regret; fear = anxiety; desire = craving or addiction; and so forth.

How we look at life is totally congruent with where we are emotionally at that moment and even the way we process life. Even the way we look at God or our creator is totally congruent with where we are in that emotional continuum as well.

On Dr. Hawkins' map of consciousness, love, joy, and inner peace are the most powerful levels associated with the most powerful emotions which lead up to enlightenment at the very top. The lowest levels on the map of consciousness are shame, guilt, and apathy, which are associated with the most weakening emotions. Courage falls somewhere in the middle, and in order for healing to start occurring, we have to be functioning at a minimum at the level of courage. Courage is correlated with empowerment. At this level, we gain the capacity to work with affirmations in order to start the healing process. At the next level, which is the level of neutrality, we start being able to let go of judgment toward ourselves and others, which is an obstacle to healing. At the level of willingness, general optimism begins to take hold. At the level of acceptance, forgiveness becomes second nature, and at the level of reason, understanding starts taking hold, which dramatically enhances our ability to heal. When we transcend reason, we gain even more traction on our healing path as we enter into the non-linear realms of existence and into the arenas of joy, love, and inner peace.

Think for a moment of the impact of these emotions on your whole being. For instance, love, joy, and peace simply do not make much sense to us when we are struggling with disease and suffering. It is hard to be rational when our inner and outer worlds are in chaos. Emotions are extremely powerful and can be very constructive, but it does take a leap of faith to generate positive emotions on a regular basis, which means we have to be able to transcend the ego and our judgments about what has happened to us in the past. Transcending the ego is a very tough thing for most human beings to accomplish because we are tied so solidly to our egos and we tend to take on more and more emotional baggage as we age.

Relationships also have a huge impact on our health, our metabolism, and our ability to lose weight and keep it off. The higher the quality of our relationships, the greater the likelihood of better emotional and physical health. We are social beings by nature, and our overall sense of well-being is closely tied to the quality of our relationships, including our relationships at home, work, and social environments. If our relationships are more ego-based we tend to harbor negative thoughts and beliefs, which tends to correlate with more negative emotions, such as hopelessness, fear, guilt, resentment, anger, and pride. In order to be successful in relationships and have them be primarily constructive and helpful towards healing, we have to gravitate toward more positive emotions in our relationships. This, of course, is much easier to accomplish when you hold more consistent, empowering belief systems.

Healthy relationships are critical for good health, and a lot of research backs up the fact that the quality of our relationships often defines our health. For example, people who are happily married are much more likely to be healthy, thin, vital, and able to heal than people who are divorced and especially those who are isolated socially. People who go to church regularly also seem more likely to heal and be healthier than people who are isolated from a church community. We are referring to any group that meets on a regular basis that meets for spiritual or religious purposes. A close-knit community is more health-promoting than being isolated.

In the same way, people who are sick and belong to support groups are healthier and heal more readily than those who are not. People who participate in constructive support groups like cancer support groups do much better than those who are isolated. In one study, cancer patients who attended regular support groups survived two to three times longer than a control group who did not attend support meetings. In a 1989 study conducted by Dr. David Spiegel at Stanford University, women with stage four metastatic breast cancer who participated in support groups lived twice as long as those who did not take part in support groups, even though all other treatments were similar. His study also found that the women in the support groups felt 50 percent less pain as the women who were not in the support groups. The women who did not belong to support groups lived an average of 19 months from the time they entered the study, but those who were in the support groups survived for an average of 36.5 months from the time they entered the study. Another study was done on patients with malignant melanomas, which are a very aggressive form of skin cancer that tend to metastasize relatively early on in the disease process. Patients who had stage four malignant melanoma and participated in support groups survived on average three times longer than patients who did not participate in the support groups.

The key principle here is when we gather together with others who are suffering from an illness but who are positive and focused on healing, that tends to empower the individual and increase their chances of healing.

Understand the Language of Your Body: What is Your Body Saying to You?

The most cost-effective medicine is getting healthy, which can only be achieved by getting to the source of an illness. The most cost-effective treatment strategies are those that discern and treat the source of the illness rather than the symptoms.

In order to treat the source of illness, we have to be able to shift our consciousness, in other words, the way we look at the world (pages 188-191 in *Heal Thyself: Transform Your Life, Transform Your Health*). We need to also understand the principles and effects of mass consciousness. For instance, in a society like the U.S., we are seeing a massive increase in the incidence of being overweight and obese in virtually every state. We are also seeing more and more people suffering from eating disorders. With four out of five adults age 25 and older classified as overweight in America today and 65 percent of all adults afflicted with the problem of being overweight, we can see that this becoming a far too common affliction. What has happened in our society is there has been a shift in mass consciousness regarding body weight.

The pandemic is characterized by unhealthy eating, the development of more chronic diseases, and progressively increasing rates of obesity and being overweight. This societal shift spans all age groups from birth to our geriatric population. In order to change our own individual outcomes, we have to start dealing with this dysfunctional mass consciousness. Let's start by challenging the belief systems held by our society as a whole, about what constitutes healthy eating and healthy living and about what is causing these exploding disease epidemics that we are facing in our society.

Sadly, even our definitions of obesity are changing. Most people that are overweight do not even see themselves as such anymore. Therefore, people often don't even realize that they have a weight problem and are surprised in many instances to be confronted with the diagnosis of obesity. The reason they feel this way is because they see themselves looking just like everyone around them! When we compare ourselves to others in our society who are also overweight and obese and fail to see enough contrast complacency settles in. The first step in healing obesity is to become conscious of what is, which does *not* mean harsh judgment, but an unemotional awakening to the facts.

The key to discovering whether we have a problem or not is to check our body weight and height against a standard body mass index (BMI) chart. Body mass index implies that we are correlating our height and weight, with a body mass index between 19 and 25 being optimal. A body mass index of 25 and above is defined as overweight, and a body mass index of 30 or above is defined as obese.

NOTE: It is also important to realize that there is much more than just your BMI score involved in defining obesity or being overweight.

Many people who are technically defined as overweight or obese are actually fit, eat healthily, have a good lean muscle mass and are just as likely or even more likely to be healthy than somebody within the ideal range who is not fit and does not eat healthily. In fact, those who are within the ideal body mass index and who are not fit or eating healthily are likely to have worse health and more health problems than those who might be classified as obese but are doing everything right. *Bringing Sexy Back* involves not condemning yourself just because of one criteria being out of range. (such as body weight or body mass index) You can be in great shape without meeting all of the ideal criteria. The premise is to love ourselves unconditionally, no matter what the numbers say.

Body mass index must be correlated with body frame. For instance, if you have a small body frame, that would correlate with a lower body mass index compared to normal range, than a large body frame, which would correlate with the higher end of the normal range. The easiest way to figure out what your body frame is to use the thumb and the middle finger of one hand to circle the wrist of your other hand at its narrowest circumference. If you can touch the thumb with the middle finger, you have a medium body frame. If you can cross those fingers, you have a small body frame, and if the two fingers cannot touch, you have a large body frame.

Another important factor to consider when evaluating weight problems is the waist-hip ratio. Someone can be overweight according to the BMI charts, but when they have an optimal waist-hip ratio, they have a relatively low likelihood of developing any health problems related to their weight. On the other hand, if the waist-hip ratio is out of normal range, even if the body mass index is ideal, they may be a higher risk for disease. To calculate the waist-hip ratio, you divide the waist measurement by the hip measurement. The ideal waist-hip ratio for a woman is 0.8 or less and for a man, 1.0 or less. A ratio greater than that means there is a substantial increase in the risk of disease for both men and women. The reason for this is because an increased waist circumference indicates more centralized obesity, which correlates with a greater number of related comorbidities. A lot of women carry extra fat around their hips with virtually no negative health implications, whereas if they carry the fat around their waist, they would be much more likely to be afflicted with health problems. We also look at actual measurements of inches around the waist and say that a waist measurement of 35 inches or less is usually associated with better health, whereas a waist measurement greater than 35 inches is associated with more serious health challenges.

It's important to look at the overall health and well-being of the person. For instance, some people have an increased BMI and increased waist measurements but absolutely no signs of physical illness. When more in-depth evaluations are done, including blood work, we may find absolutely no signs of abnormality. If their blood sugars are optimal, their cholesterol or lipid panels are in the optimal range, and no signs of any health problems, including blood pressure, joint problems, back problems, and so forth, then it may mean that their obesity does not have any immediate significance to their health. When we refer back to Recall

Healing, it makes it easier to understand why some people have frank obesity but are otherwise absolutely healthy, whereas others who are absolutely normal in terms of their body weight have dire health challenges. We should avoid the temptation to jump to conclusions based on one set of criteria about someone's health.

Don't do it.

Integrating Thoughts, Energy, Lifestyle, and Physiology

Empowering beliefs and positive emotions are essential for overall good health and are also associated with positive thoughts, increased energy, and a much easier time controlling lifestyle and improving physiology. By examining our beliefs, rooting out those beliefs that are disempowering and by taking on more empowering belief systems, we achieve a major positive impact on our overall health. One of the tools we use to turn around dysfunctional belief systems is positive affirmations, which help reprogram the mind and clear out negative thoughts that are having a negative impact on our health.

There are seven empowering beliefs that are essential for healing. They are:

1. The belief that you *can* be healed.

2. The belief that you *will* be healed.

3. The belief that you *deserve* to be healed.

4. The *belief* in miracles.

5. The belief that we are subject *only* to what we hold in mind.

6. The belief that we are infinite beings with *infinite capacity* to heal.

7. Healing is as simple as *discovering* and *repairing* the unresolved conflicts that programmed us for our illness.

For example, it is critical that we have a very strong and unbending belief that you can take weight off and keep it off. Many people don't believe that they can take the weight off. Even if they believe they can lose weight, they do not believe, deep down, that they can keep it off. This is especially true when they have been unsuccessful numerous times in the past in their attempts. Even one failure to lose weight and/or keep it off can engrain a disempowering belief and doom you to endless cycles of failure.

Many people believe they can take the weight off if they do the right thing, but they have a deep-seated skepticism that they personally will be unable to succeed. They have seen other people succeed and absolutely believe *other* people can do it, but some people have a doubt about having the strength of character or the spirit to do so themselves. Oftentimes, it is related to their past failures to lose weight, keep it off, and control the cravings.

A lot of people also have deep-seated belief systems that make them feel, at least at a subconscious level, that they don't necessarily deserve to be thin. Sometimes those beliefs correspond with their religious faith, and many of us suffer from deep-seated guilt complexes that may make us believe that our weight issue is just punishment from God for past sins. If you don't believe that you deserve to be thin or to be healed from your affliction, this will most certainly block your ability to succeed.

A lot of people have the belief that in order to be successful with weight loss and keeping weight off, they need tremendous levels of willpower, which they don't believe they have. Most people just don't believe that there are any easy solutions, and they certainly don't see the possibility of miraculous healing taking place. And yet, when you talk to people who have been successful with losing weight and keeping it off long term, they often relay the idea that their weight loss was nearly effortless and even miraculous. As a matter of fact, you rarely hear of someone who was successful in losing weight and keeping it off through sheer willpower. The use of willpower to lose weight and keep it off means that you have not found the key or the emotional root to your weight problem.

People who are successful with long-term weight will often claim that some kind of major shift happened within them to dramatically change the way they live their lives. As we learn more about Recall Healing and understand the roots of illness, we will be able to generate revelations that shed massive light on why we gained so much weight in the first place. This is the foundation for bringing about massive healing. But it all starts with the key belief that miracles can happen for you in your efforts to heal what, for most, is a longstanding and often extremely frustrating and overwhelming problem.

Arthur C. Clarke wrote, "Miracles happen not in opposition to nature, but in opposition to what we *know* of nature." After all, life itself is a miracle, and every moment of our lives is spent healing from something, even if it is just something like a scrape or a cut.

Albert Einstein also believed in miracles. He once said, "There are only two ways to live your life. One is as though there are no miracles, and the other is as though everything is a miracle." Here is where we can look at not just the possibility, but the fact that even obesity is miraculous if we understand the purpose and meaning of it. Why does obesity occur? What is the solution to the deeper, biological dilemma? As a matter of fact, we can get a sense of the miraculous when we look at obesity as absolutely essential for the survival of the individual at the time they developed it. Believing in miracles becomes incredibly powerful when we truly understand what miracles are, how to allow for them, bring them about more routinely and recognize them.

The fifth essential empowering belief is the fact that we are subject only to what we hold in our mind. We need to realize that thoughts are things and that we literally create our realities with the thoughts we hold onto in terms of our inner and outer realities. When we hold a lot of negative thoughts and beliefs in mind, it correlates with a very troublesome, painful, and disease-ridden reality. Our thoughts are then fortified by what we experience and see in our outer universe, which in turn causes further manifestation of disease and pain because of our focus on the negative. This becomes a vicious cycle that most of us live with pretty much on a consistent basis.

For instance, when we look at ourselves in the mirror and judge ourselves to be ugly or unattractive, that correlates with a very negative self-image of ourselves, which makes it virtually impossible to change our metabolisms or to change our destinies in terms of our body weight. However, when we break the cycle of misery and start having thoughts that are aligned with thinness and we start getting excited about being thin and accomplishing thinness, that totally changes the energy that runs through our bodies. In other words, when we shift our thoughts toward greater empowerment and wellness, healing and losing weight become far more achievable.

You can literally think yourself thin.

Number six on this list is the belief that we are infinite beings with an infinite capacity to heal. This belief is related to our quantum physical nature, which is linked with the concept of infinity and the fact that our energy fields extend from our bodies into infinity. We are much more than just a physical body. We are energy beings with a spiritual aspect that may also need healing. It becomes easier to heal and lose weight when we understand the fact that we are infinite beings and that we are linked with an infinite wisdom.

The seventh essential empowering belief is recognizing that unresolved conflicts programmed us for our conditions like obesity or eating disorders and that resolving and clearing these conflicts are essential to healing the problem. In order to clear the problem, we have to name it, claim it, and dump it.

Sal Landeros, two-time Fred Astaire National Champion in Ball Room Dancing, lost over 47 pounds. He went from 234 pounds to 185 pounds, although his weight was as high as 250 pounds before he started seeing me. His weight finally settled at 195 pounds where he is most comfortable and feels the healthiest, and he has been able to maintain his weight at this level. He has also been able to reverse his hypertension, high cholesterol, and high triglycerides without medicines or supplements. In other words, he reduced his risk for cardiovascular disease, which runs in his family, and has a lot more energy to boot. He worked through a lot of emotional blocks to get where he is today.

###

I have been in Dr. De Wet's care off and on for the past several years. In all, I've lost about 38 pounds, and it took me just seven weeks to lose that. Dr. De Wet put me on the modified fast initially and eventually moved me up to the Green Life Diet, phase one, by gradually adding certain food choices. For instance, relatively early on I went from just eating vegetables and fruits mainly with some nuts and seeds to adding a little bit of steak or chicken a couple times a week in small portions. Most of the time I eat salads and other green vegetables like spinach and green beans. I also eat a lot of fruit. I keep something healthy to snack on so that I am eating about every four hours. The first seven days I did that, I lost about seven pounds. The next thing I knew, I just kept losing it and losing. I also do a lot of walking and exercise at least an hour a day.

*I was about 238 pounds when I first went to see Dr. De Wet, and I got down to 185 pounds, but I felt like that made me too skinny. I discovered that the average weight that looked good for me and that I felt very good at was between 195 and 200, especially taking into account that I exercise a whole lot and am extremely active as a ballroom dance teacher and carry more muscle mass than average. I felt and looked good. I went from a size 40 pants to a size 34. I had this dance shirt, which I've had for 22 years, and **I outgrew it**. One day I saw it hanging up in the closet and was getting ready to go to a competition and wondered if I would be able to get into it. I certainly did, and with room to spare!*

When I was young and slim, I used to wear that shirt often, but it had probably been a good 17 years since I was able to fit into it, and it was very snug toward the end. It's a really nice white shirt with piano notes on the collar, and every time I wear it, I get nothing but compliments about it.

I originally went to see Dr. De Wet for a fungus issue on my toenails and fingernails, so that initial visit had nothing to do with my weight. He put me on a detox regimen to cleanse my body, and through that I started to lose the weight as well as the fungus. It just cleaned out and purified my system, and now I continue to do this with the Green Life Diet. I learned the importance of natural products because of how well the body processes them compared to conventional drugs. For example, I found out things such as butter is healthier than margarine, and I've eliminated margarine completely from my diet.

When I first went to see Dr. De Wet, I had high cholesterol and high blood pressure. I was also worried about diabetes and heart disease because I have both of these running in my family. I just knew that I had all of these things going against me in spite of taking care of myself the best I could.

Dr. De Wet taught me how to control my weight, when I can cheat and when I can't cheat. This has made it much easier for me to keep the weight off for the long term. In the past, I tried to lose weight, but I always starved myself and would end up putting it back on in just a few weeks. Eventually I gave up and decided that it was a waste of time, but this time I stuck with the Green Life Diet because I saw results immediately and knew that it would be better for my health.

In addition to the diet, Dr. De Wet also used a special IV (chelation) to clean out (detox) heavy metals that affecting my (cardiovascular) system. It made my whole body feel warm inside. I also took supplements to replenish my body because during the detox process, nutrients were also getting flushed out, so I had to replenish them by taking supplements.

Overall, I am much healthier than I have been in a long time. Everyone who knew me said I looked great. I've been doing professional ballroom dancing for a long time, and it feels good to put on some nice pants and know that I look just as good as these 20-year-olds I'm competing against. I'm in my 50s now, so it is just great that I can put something that's nice fitting on and feel comfortable going up against these young guys.

The biggest challenge I experienced throughout this whole

process was being disciplined. I didn't cheat at all, even when I would go out with my wife and she would have a few drinks and I would stick to my healthy eating plan. That was the hardest thing, to stick with it when everyone around me was having what I couldn't have. But I found out that you can go out and have a good time without drinking a lot or even drinking anything at all. I drink water instead.

If you're serious about losing weight, then you'll make the changes, but if you're not serious about losing weight, then you will tend to cheat and the next thing you know, you will be back to where you were. It all depends on what you want to get out of it.

Chapter Four:

A Layman's Guide to a Doctor's World: Understanding Fat Physiology

"There is not a single drug on the market today that doesn't have some negative impact on our health; regardless of the justification for its use."

—Dr. Pieter De Wet

In this chapter we will be discussing different characteristics of fat including its specific physiological functions. Fat plays many roles in the human body from a physiological and emotional perspective. We discovered the emotional perspectives in our previous chapters. For example, fat acts as a container in the body for fat-soluble toxins, thereby reducing the negative impacts of these toxins on critical structures within the body, such as the brain and cardiovascular system. Fat also acts as an insulator, keeping body heat in while keeping cold out—in other words, protecting us against temperature extremes in the winter. Fat also acts as a flotation device because fat, after all, is lighter than water, so it actually helps the body to be more buoyant when immersed in water. Fat is also a critical source of energy, and is most intimately linked with survival of the body in times of scarcity or when starvation sets in. Fat can also be framed as a huge hormonal gland because it makes numerous hormones and metabolizes numerous others.

There are numerous other hormonal glands in the body, neurotransmitters produced by the brain, and numerous other structures in the human body that play critical roles in regulating metabolism. Hormones are an often overlooked physiological system that is critical to understand in order to attain optimal weight and health. Ignoring their importance will sidetrack any effort to improve health, shed excess fat and boost metabolism. Let's take a look at how hormones work.

Hormone Basics

There are a series of hormones that play a very critical role in our physiology as it relates to metabolism. These include adrenal hormones, thyroid hormones, sex hormones, hormones related to sugar metabolism, digestion, and fat metabolism. There are even hormones produced during pregnancy that can have dramatic effects on metabolism.

Testosterone

Testosterone is critical for the development and maintenance of strong muscles in the body, including the heart muscle, as well as the skeletal muscles. Skeletal muscles are critical to maintaining healthy metabolism because of the calories they burn, not just during activity, but at rest. The greater your muscle mass, the greater the amount of calories you burn, even at rest, and the greater your capacity to exercise and thereby increase your calorie burning even more dramatically. Testosterone is also associated with levels of energy and even personality characteristics such as creativity and assertiveness. Most people who are not creative lack assertiveness, proactiveness, and willpower. These are all critical characteristics that need to be developed if not already present if one wants to succeed in losing weight and maintaining it. Testosterone is not just critical in men, but in women, as well. In both men and women it is also associated with sex drive and bone strength. Engaging in more sex is correlated with better metabolism and maintaining a healthy body weight. Another great way to bring sexy back!

Adrenal Hormones

The adrenal glands produce certain key hormones that are also critical in maintaining optimal energy and metabolism. DHEA, for example, is a critical hormone that we need at optimal levels in order to maintain energy. It is also a biomarker of biological age and correlates with longevity. If your DHEA levels are low, prematurely depleted or decreased, then it is often an indicator of premature biological aging beyond your chronological age. This also correlated with fatigue problems. Of course, when you are more prone to fatigue, then you are less likely to exercise and more prone to engage in behaviors that will artificially increase energy production. This includes the ingestion of sugary or starchy foods and the consumption of other stimulants, such as caffeine and even street drugs such as amphetamines.

There are other adrenal hormones that are also important for energy production and for controlling inflammation in the body. These include cortisol, hydrocortisone, and androstenedione. Hydrocortisone and cortisol are critical hormones to reduce inflammation in the body and increasing energy production. On the other hand, they can also be a problem when overproduced or when administered externally, especially in synthetic form (prednisone, dexamethasone, betamethasone). These natural anti-inflammatory hormones are critical in the healing of injured tissues, such as muscles, joints, and ligaments, that occur when exercising vigorously. Excessive production of these stress hormones (cortisol and hydrocortisone) or the use of synthetic corticosteroids from external sources tends to contribute to obesity.

Cushing's Syndrome

Cushing's syndrome is an internal production problem (when the adrenals overproduce cortisol). This is characterized by central obesity with relatively thin extremities in contrast to severe stretch marks on the abdomen, a moon face, and often a dysfunctional immune system as well. We also see these very same symptoms in people treated with corticosteroids, including synthetic steroids, for diseases such as autoimmune diseases, asthma, allergies, pain in the joints, back and neck pain, etc.

There are many other hormones also involved in fat metabolism, and we'll discuss a few more in this upcoming section. It is important to note though that virtually all hormones produced in our bodies affect body weight in some way, shape, or form, either directly or indirectly. When any hormonal system in the body is out of balance, it can affect our physiology and, therefore, contribute to obesity or a resistance to weight loss. Whenever a patient with obesity and other very serious health problems comes into my office, we test certain hormone levels, through blood, saliva, urine or bio-energetic data collection methods (using bio-energetic technologies such as EAV electro-acupuncture by Voll technology). Hormonal workups for those with dysfunctional metabolisms may include thyroid and adrenal hormones and some or all of the following hormones:

1. **Insulin** – regulates the metabolism of carbohydrates but indirectly contributes to fattening. Insulin resistance is a major factor for those who suffer with obesity and the other health problems that typically go along with it, such as diabetes, hypertension, hyperlipidemia, cancer, and heart disease. Insulin contributes to fattening indirectly because it triggers the cells in the body to take up more sugar into them, which then has to be converted to fat molecules for longer term storage. The more insulin resistant you become, the more insulin the pancreas has to make in order to process

the same amount of sugar coming from food sources such as starches, grains, and so forth.

2. **Leptin** – a hormone produced by fat. When we consume processed foods they eventually go into storage in the fat tissues. The fat tissues, in turn, produce a hormone called leptin, which works at the level of the hypothalamus to suppress appetite. Leptin increases when fat cells are full in order to signal the brain to reduce appetite and thereby reduce calorie intake. Sometimes people who are obese have leptin resistance, which is similar to insulin resistance. People who have insulin resistance typically develop leptin resistance.

3. **Ghrelin** – this hormone has the opposite effect of leptin and is responsible for stimulation of appetite. This is another hormone that is released by fat tissue when we are not consuming enough calories. When we are trying to lose weight, we should make every effort to keep this hormone level low. The most important method to reduce production of ghrelin is to eat more frequently, so when we eat five or six more meals a day, for example, it helps to suppress the production of ghrelin. In contrast it becomes nearly impossible to control ghrelin production when we only eat once or twice a day.

4. **Cholecystokinin** – this hormone's primary purpose is the suppression of appetite. It is manufactured by the first part of the small bowel just outside of the stomach and gets released in response to fat consumption. This is one reason why low fat diets

don't make *any* sense because when you eat a diet that is low in fat, your small bowel will produce more cholecystokinin which drives your brain to crave foods that have more fat in them. It is much better, therefore, to eat a diet rich in healthy fats. According to scientific data, there is no evidence that fat consumption makes us fat. As a matter of fact, fat is critical to health. It is a key element in optimal function of your brain and the production of hormones that are critical for maintaining optimal metabolism. Every meal of the day should include significant amounts of healthy fats as part of it. We will discuss what those healthy fats are in a later chapter.

5. **DHEA** and **17-keto DHEA** – as we mentioned earlier, an energy hormone. Another hormone called 17-keto DHEA is related to DHEA and is also another very important hormone that's very helpful for boosting metabolism and improving our ability to lose weight.

6. **βHCG** – the hormone produced in women when they are pregnant and more specifically, produced by the placenta in order to ensure a constant supply of nutrients to the fetus throughout pregnancy. This hormone is unique. It is the single most effective tool that I know to liberate fat from pathological fat stores in the body. It is literally like a lock and key system that very efficiently causes the body to burn pathological fat while simultaneously ensuring the maintenance of life itself (which is why pregnant

women require it). βHCG also ensures the body will not access vital fat stores such as structural fat in the brain and nervous system, subcutaneous fat critical for protection against temperature extremes, and the fat surrounding critical organs that acts as a cushion against trauma. βHCG ensures protection of protein stores in the body, such as those in the muscles and connective tissues that are critical in giving the body its form, including skin, bones, ligaments and tendons.

β HCG ensures that the body will not access these tissues and other organs to replace the calories needed in order to keep the body alive when going on calorie restrictions associated with an effort to lose weight. β HCG gives both men and women the same advantage in terms of weight loss as it does during pregnancy by giving us the ability to access pathological fat stores and burn up that fat preferentially. It also gives us a much better ability to maintain that weight loss over the long term. This also occurs because of the resetting effect of the β HCG on the hypothalamic fat metabolism control center. Even though β HCG is effective for both men and women, men tend to lose weight more easily on β HCG than women do. For example, the average adult male can lose, on average, about 31 pounds per 42 days on β HCG, whereas a woman on average can lose about 22 pounds during a 42 day course of β HCG.

NOTE: For those of you interested in using β HCG for weight loss, the following precautions must be observed. Dr. Simeon's HCG protocol has been used for the last

40+ years for effective and safe weight loss. His protocol must be followed *meticulously* when using β HCG.

The β HCG has come into disrepute of late because of unscrupulous companies trying to sell massive amounts of homeopathic β HCG promising unreasonable amounts of weight loss and giving very little if any guidance as to how to proceed safely with the very low calorie diet (VLC) supported by β HCG. The biggest mistake people make when using a β HCG diet is to restrict their caloric intake to less than the 500 calories per day. The second biggest mistake is continuing longer than is recommended (beyond 42 days, including the two days of fat loading).

For more information on the Simeon protocol, go to my website at www.qhiwellness.com. Go to shopqui.com and click on the weight loss package with β HCG. There you will find Dr. Simeon's 70-page protocol.

The Consequences of Big Pharma

What effect do pharmaceuticals have on our health and metabolism? We've already discussed the role hormones play with our body's metabolism. The fact is, hormones are naturally occurring in the body and sometimes can be replenished from outside, (β HCG, for example). This would support the idea that pharmaceutical intervention can speed up metabolism. On the other hand, synthetic hormones (in fact, ALL drugs) that are manufactured by pharmaceutical companies can and almost always do have unintended consequences. The reason this occurs is because drugs treat symptoms, not causes and in turn they cause side effects or more disease. What the pharmaceutical industry is selling is the concept that we can *cure* illnesses by *managing* symptoms.

This is ludicrous.

You cannot heal a disease by shooting the messenger. Not only is this un-physiological, but massive corruption has made its way into our health care system because of the influence the pharmaceutical industry wields over the prescribing habits of health care providers. The pharmaceutical industry's exorbitant profits not only affect our health care system, but our political system. The health insurance industry is more than happy to pay for very expensive pharmaceuticals that do little more than treat symptoms and refuse to pay for those treatments that have the potential to prevent or reverse illness.

There is no financial incentive to cure anything.

Conventional pharmaceuticals create unintended side effects, including weight gain due to the impairment of metabolism. Another common side effect of many pharmaceuticals is fatigue, which in turn contributes to weight gain because of the resultant reluctance to exercise. It is a never ending spiral of doing the wrong thing for the right reason.

There is a long list of other direct and indirect side effects associated with most drugs that also have adverse impacts on metabolism and, therefore, increase the likelihood of weight gain. These include effects such as:

- Sleep problems

- Loss of stamina
- Decreased muscle strength
- Adrenal stress
- Negative impacts on pituitary function
- Brain fog or effects on brain physiology

Additionally, if a drug is fat soluble, it dissolves into our fat tissues and makes it very difficult to get rid of that fat. The body will not give up fat soluble toxins very readily due to adverse impacts on critical structures such as the brain and cardiovascular system. As a result, we are much more likely to accumulate more fat when taking pharmaceuticals that are fat soluble in order to act as a buffer against those toxins.

There is not a single drug on the market today that doesn't have some negative impact on our health, no matter what the justification for its use is in the first place. By treating symptoms, you are essentially suppressing the body's own protective mechanisms and the body's indicators that show you that something has gone wrong or is out of balance. You're denying the message your body is giving you instead of trying to figure out what the message means.

It never pays to treat just the symptoms.

When you get to the root of the problem, you can dramatically correct what is going wrong, often in a very short amount of time by giving the body the nutrients it needs and by removing the obstacles to healing. It is very seldom that we actually need to take pharmaceutical or prescription drugs. There are certainly exceptions.

Conventional medicine is great in terms of removing certain threats to immediate survival, for instance, when someone has a severely elevated blood pressure or blood sugar. In cases such as these, we may need to prescribe and have someone take a drug to counter that crisis for a short period of time. Certainly, in emergency situations such as heart attacks or other life-threatening emergencies we want the best life-saving drugs to be used. But, even in many emergencies there are natural solutions that can be very helpful in addition to pharmaceuticals.

Bad Drugs! Understanding Drugs and Drug Categories

Of course there are many different categories of drugs, and there are certainly some drug categories that are far worse than others, especially in terms of obesity. These drug categories are great contributors to the obesity epidemic facing us today:

1. **Antidepressants:** Virtually every antidepressant on the market except for one (bupropion, which is marketed under the name brand Wellbutrin) has negative effects on metabolism. Most antidepressants also increase insulin resistance, and therefore increase the risk of diabetes, high cholesterol, high triglycerides, and hypertension.

2. **Antipsychotics:** Most antipsychotic drugs have an adverse impact on metabolism and contribute to

obesity by stimulating appetite, increasing fatigue, and slowing metabolism.

3. **Insomnia drugs:** All drugs used for insomnia slow down metabolism indirectly through their negative impact on sleep rhythms. Even though the drug makes you feel like you are sleeping more, it causes the quality of your sleep to deteriorate. The result is more fatigue, which contributes to habits that are not conducive to weight loss.

4. **Anti-diabetes drugs:** Sulfonylurea (including glipizide and glyburide) cause weight gain by directly or indirectly increasing insulin levels in the body. Even as they reduce sugar levels, they ultimately increase the risk of more diabetes by driving body weight upwards. As far as diabetes drugs go, there are a couple of exceptions to the rule. There are two drug categories that specifically don't increase the likelihood of weight gain but actually can contribute to weight loss, and those include metformin, which tends to be a more favorable drug as far as helping people gain control of their weight, and byetta, which is made from Gila monster saliva and tends to suppress appetite and contribute to weight loss. The latter drug, byetta, has a high incidence of adverse effects on the gastrointestinal tract within six months of starting it, with very few people being able to tolerate the drug for more than a year or two.

5. **Narcotics and other painkillers:** These drugs affect our energy, gut functions, liver, and other

organs in the body, which indirectly or directly contribute to obesity. Narcotics also have specific adverse effects on waste elimination, including a tendency to cause constipation. This, of course makes it difficult to optimize metabolism. These drugs, especially the narcotics, affect our mindsets and cause problems with motivation in those trying to implement healthier lifestyles.

Whenever you are given a prescription for a drug or pharmaceutical, the very first question you should ask your physician should be about side effects. Don't restrict your questions to the side effects listed on the label, either. Ask about *unlisted* side effects that people complain about. It is also a good idea to do some online research to see what other people are saying about the drug that you're about to begin taking. A good doctor will ask patients what kinds of side effects they are experiencing, so they will know what additional side effects these drugs can cause. Unfortunately the FDA does not require companies to list every side effect, especially those that are more non-specific, like weight gain, fatigue, sleep problems, etc.

Vicky Brannon lost over 20 pounds. She went from 156 pounds to 136 pounds and went down four pants sizes. She now manages her hypertension without medicines or supplements. Her energy was much better; she reversed age-related changes of her skin. She also reversed her chronic bladder infections and other problems, including problems with emotional well-being.

###

When I went to see Dr. De Wet, I lost over 21 pounds in just 40 days. I started at 156 pounds and went down to 134. I also had high cholesterol, and that went down as well. Both my husband and I benefited from Dr. De Wet's knowledge and care. We were both placed on Dr. De Wet's β HCG weight loss program, which involves eating just 500 calories a day and using the β HCG to stimulate metabolism, as well as a couple of other supplement combinations to further optimize metabolism, appetite control, and bowel function. My husband actually lost 25 pounds, going from 180 down to 155. He is a double amputee who is in a wheelchair, and the extra weight was affecting his shoulders and his wrists severely, so it was very beneficial for him to lose the weight as well.

I didn't become a research scientist or anything. However, Dr. De Wet isn't a doctor who simply gives you a remedy and instructions. He places a strong emphasis on educating and empowering his patients. I have not only made huge strides in my health, I've learned so much, I could probably teach a weight loss class to others!

I was using the β HCG cream and working directly with Dr. De Wet and my husband was using the β HCG homeopathic spray, which he ordered through Dr. De Wet's website and was able to use that without having to see a physician in a clinic environment (we worked under Dr. De Wet's supervision through his weekly tele-support group). I think my husband had a bit of an advantage because I just used the β HCG cream once in the morning, and he used the β HCG homeopathic spray up to six times a day. That seemed to help him with the hunger pangs. I think my problem was more psychological because he seemed to be able to be more proactive with his more frequent use of the spray.

I had high cholesterol and high blood pressure, but both of those problems were reversed without medications. One of the reasons I first started seeing Dr. De Wet was because in the past, I had been allergic to almost any treatments I received. I was sensitive to most medications, so I was scared of them. In fact, I had minor surgery, which required me to receive just 5 milligrams of valium, and it actually stopped my heart on the table and I had to be resuscitated (brought back to life). I'm very thankful for natural products such as those that Dr. De Wet prescribes.

As a 61-year-old, I needed guidance with these things because I was on statin drugs for cholesterol, but they made me sick because they weakened my muscles and caused problems with my memory. I tried to diet and exercise, but it didn't work. I was impressed with Dr. De Wet because he's not just a medical doctor, which is important because he's educated in conventional medicine, but he also uses alternative routes of treatment to help.

When he started telling me about the β HCG weight loss program, I knew that I would have been crazy to jump on it without his care. But I think having a doctor watching over me just added to the success and the feeling that I could do it because he was supervising me. We had weekly telephone support groups that we participated in, which I was thankful for because I felt like I could be missing something without a doctor to answer questions (this included questions about Dr. De Wet's β HCG weight loss program *both through his clinic in Tyler called QHI Wellness and through his website at www.shopqhi.com.) Dr. De Wet also went public with his own dieting success to encourage his patients and listeners, which is also very helpful to me and my husband and inspired us to start the program. Dr. De Wet lost 40 pounds in 42 days, which impressed us to the point where we decided to do it as well.*

The idea behind the β HCG weight loss program is that you use the β HCG hormone multiple times a day if you're doing the homeopathic spray and you only eat 500 calories a day. It sounds crazy, but this hormone keeps you from being hungry. It's the hormone that your body secretes when you are pregnant, but the body then releases stored fat and starts burning it because of the hormone.

In working with Dr. De Wet, I also went through Recall Healing workshops with him to help me understand what the root causes were of my weight issues and help me become more proactive with those particular conflicts programming me for obesity. There were a couple of times during my weight loss program where my weight loss stopped (I hit two plateaus), but when I confronted the emotional root linked with those plateaus, I was able to resolve them and break through with my weight loss so that I could get further down with my weight. Dr. De Wet was very helpful in guiding me through those particular plateaus. In Dr. De Wet's Book, Heal Thyself: Transform Your Life, Transform Your Health, *he has also listed the conflicts programming for obesity, and the book was very helpful in reminding me what I was working through in order to be more successful long-term.*

The most fascinating thing for me was I've been on Weight Watchers before and tried the β HCG Diet before. (Which failed to work) Even with the limited weight loss that I achieved, it came straight back. While I was doing Dr. De Wet's HCG program, he encouraged me to keep a written record of what I weighed each day and every time I got stuck on a weight or hit a plateau, he asked me to go back and figure out exactly when in my life I was at that weight and asked me to remember the emotions that were associated with that time in my life and that particular weight, like for instance when my daughter's home was destroyed and she moved back in with us, causing some stress in the household related to her future, which looked somewhat bleak at that point. It also had to do with an invasion of territory, which was, of course, experienced at the subconscious level. We love our daughter, but having an adult move in with grandkids in tow can be somewhat stressful as anyone can imagine, especially if you don't know for how long that was going to be the case.

It has been much easier to keep the weight off this time. My weight only fluctuated four pounds from my lowest weight, and this was after several weeks on vacation starting with a trip to France. I walked a lot on this vacation, so that also helped. I could almost eat whatever I wanted when I was walking so much. But I found that it's easier to behave when I have emotional support and have dealt with the problems that are at the roots of my weight loss. At this point I am not back on the diet, but it's easier to say that I've accomplished this weight loss with greater insight into the breakthroughs that it took to get there and will watch what I'm going to do from now on. That will include walking more and cutting out the unhealthy snacks that contributed to my weight gain previously.

Each week when I would call in for the conference call, I would write something about the week. The first week of the call, I wrote, "In my 60 plus years, I've been on every diet you can imagine, even bananas. I have had to shop for strange foods. I have had to plan, measure, find recipes, and learn to cook strange things. All of these programs gave me success for only a short period of time. But what I love about the β HCG program is that it's not about the food. It's like a vacation from all of the complexity described above."

On the β HCG program, I would spend one day each week gathering the fruits and vegetables that I would need for the week. By day 27, I had lost 12 pounds and 11 inches. I am grateful to have participated in this diet. I ate nothing for breakfast, and I would start the day at lunch with one serving of vegetables, 100 grams of protein, and one breadstick. At supper I would repeat that. The nice thing is the entire program is described in full in the information I received from Dr. De Wet's office and that my husband received from the Internet when he ordered his β HCG protocol from Dr. De Wet's website. It was easy and straightforward and has led to ultimate success.

Chapter Five:
Body Rehab: Removing Obstacles to Great Metabolism

"Exercise is not a dirty word. With increased physical movement, you not only burn calories, but increase joint flexibility, circulation and your quality of life."

—Dr. Pieter De Wet

Every habit we have potentially impacts our health.

Even our habits relating to our environment has a direct impact on our health. Where we spend our time and what we allow ourselves to be exposed to defines our health in many ways, including our metabolism. For example, people who spend a lot of time in nature, whether it is related to their job or a hobby, tend to have better metabolisms than those who spend a lot of time indoors. People who are indoors most of the time are usually in front of a television set or doing sedentary activities like sitting in front of a computer. Several studies have shown correlations between, the amount of television that we watch and the incidence of and levels of obesity, both in children and in adults.

There are plenty of things we can do to transform our environment so that we will be more likely to thrive. Even if we work in an office for 10 or 12 hours a day, there are small adjustments that we can make to reduce the negative impact of certain environmental factors on our bodies. Here are 19 obvious, but often overlooked steps we can take to remove obstacles to achieve great metabolism.

1. **More time outdoors.**

Being outside usually translates to more physical, calorie-burning activities. We are much more likely to spend time walking, lifting, pushing, pulling, gardening, playing with your children, running around, etc.—all activities that increase our calorie burning—than we are when we are indoors. Get outside. Go for a walk. Move. Feel better and burn more calories.

2. **Get more sun.**

Spending more time outside speeds up our metabolism for many reasons. More sun exposure typically translates into a faster metabolism because exposure to sunlight increases our body's manufacturing and activation of vitamin D3, which reduces inflammation in your body. There's a clear correlation between vitamin D3 deficiency and increased incidence of obesity. The common pathway is inflammation because vitamin D3 deficiency is associated with increased incidence of inflammation, which is primarily what obesity represents in the body. Even when we can't spend a lot of time outdoors to get more sun exposure, we can open blinds and windows indoors to let more sunlight indoors, directly or indirectly, which has a positive impact on both moods and body rhythms. This will result in better sleep cycles and circadian rhythms (adrenal-cortisol production cycles).

More people are living under the false impression that sunlight is dangerous for us and should be avoided, almost at all cost.

This simply is not true.

Excessive sun exposure can certainly cause skin damage, but this is blown way out of proportion compared to what the real risks are. The result is that most people are getting inadequate sun exposure and vitamin D3 deficiency is becoming an epidemic in our society, with seriously impacts not just metabolism, but numerous other critical body functions.

3. **Optimize the benefits and minimize the damage from the sun.**

Everyone should be exposed to direct sunlight every day if at all possible unless they have some severe skin disease that makes them hyper-sensitive to sun exposure. Exposure to direct sunlight is better than exposure to indirect sunlight (either indoors through windows or outdoors in the shadows), although there are benefits to both. Direct sunlight is not only good for you because of the activation of vitamin D to D3, it also optimizes moods, reduces depression, optimizes immune system function, etc. The most optimal time to get sun exposure is midday. The amount of time spent in sunshine should be 20 to 30 minutes at noon at full sun with at least 60 percent of the body exposed if you are light skinned. The darker your skin, the more time you need in direct sun in order to get the same benefits. Remember, during the winter months it is nearly impossible to get enough direct sun for activation of D3, unless you live closer to the equator. It is therefore critical for most people to take extra D3 as a supplement. This is especially true for those who are unlikely to get adequate sun and for those with darker skin.

Most of the commercial suntan lotions with artificial ingredients give us a false sense of security and may do more harm than good. The reason for this unintended harm is because the lotions filter out the UVB rays very well but not the UVA rays. It is the UVA fraction of the ultraviolet spectrum that is linked with an increased incidence of skin cancer, whereas UVB rays are the rays that cause the activation of vitamin D to D3. Certain types of suntan lotions and sun-blocks are better alternatives for skin protection for those who spend a lot of time outdoors and who need to protect especially sensitive areas of skin. Zinc-based sunblock is good for protection of sensitive areas of the skin like the nose and the lower eyelids against UVA and UVB rays.

Contact our clinic at www.qhiwellness.com for a comprehensive list of supplements including D3 and others.

4. Appropriate clothing protects the skin much better than toxic chemicals.

There is a lot of clothing specifically-rated for sun protection, and certain materials are well-known to be more protective than others. Jeans and khaki are a couple examples of materials that give good protection from the sun. Instead of trying to cover up with suntan lotions, it is often better just to protect yourself with clothes if you're going to be out in the sun for extended periods of time. That includes head protection with appropriately-sized hats that protect not just the facial skin but the neck. As mentioned before, a good amount of the body should be exposed for at least some time every day in order to get proper activation of Vitamin D, but outside of that we should cover up properly or stay out of the sun if possible. The toxic chemicals in most suntan lotions can contribute to slowing down your metabolism and may be carcinogenic.

The Toxic Price of Beautification

5. Avoid makeup that is full of toxins.

A very common source for major toxicity in the human body, especially in women, comes from the cosmetics they use on their skin. Nearly all makeup is full of toxic chemicals that can adversely impact metabolism. In the U.S., rules governing the typical ingredients in cosmetics tend to be very lax, especially when compared to other countries like those in Europe. This is of grave concern. The golden rule is that you should never put anything on your skin that you wouldn't be willing to consume by mouth. Therefore, when using cosmetics, it is critical to use options that are made up of naturally occurring ingredients. 'Organic' and 'natural' are two of the keywords that you want to look for when purchasing cosmetics. More and more women are also voting with their feet and not purchasing as many cosmetics as before, which may be good for their health and their pocketbooks. Many cosmetics contain sunblock and sunscreen, which also add to the toxicity of these products and give a false sense of security in terms of protection against sun damage.

The Obsession with Artificial Intelligence

Every piece of electrical technology around us emits a field of electromagnetic interference (called electro-smog) to a greater or lesser extent. Some devices have minimal impact, while others have potentially more severe impact that can be even catastrophic to our health and metabolism over the long-term when exposed to on a daily basis.

6. Limit your exposure to radiation from electronic devices.

We all live in an era where electronic devices form an integral part of everyday life. These devices emit electromagnetic frequency (EMF). For most of us, it is hard to imagine functioning without these devices. In fact, electronic devices can overwhelm us and consume us if we aren't mindful. What few people seem to be aware of is the actual adverse health impacts that we incur when we spend too much time near these devices.

There seems to be a strong correlation between the amount of time we spend consumed with our electronic devices and the incidence of obesity and sluggish metabolism. Not only is it affecting our adult population, but it's having massive negative impacts on our children when they become consumed with electronic devices, such as televisions, computers, gaming devices, etc. We see our children spending more time sitting in the school classroom behind a computer and then coming home and sitting in front of a television, gaming device or computer. This lifestyle is one of the primary drivers of the obesity epidemic in our children starting at younger and younger ages. Adults and children should find a better balance, spending more time away from these devices and outdoors or find innovative ways to combine these devices with activity. The gaming industry is making it possible to do so with more and more games for gaming consoles focused on increasing physical activity.

These electronic devices (through EMF) have an indirect negative impact by causing us to be more sedentary and spend more time indoors. Additionally, they can also have a direct negative impact on metabolism by disturbing communication between cells and by affecting cell function. Devices that have the greatest potential for negative impact on inter-cellular communication include cordless phones and Wi-Fi network devices. Unfortunately in virtually every work place, hotel, shop, and in most homes now, we are getting exposed to large doses of Wi-Fi radiation. One of the worst places in the world to be is in an apartment complex where you might be surrounded by dozens and dozens of other Wi-Fi devices in other apartments around you.

Wi-Fi, cordless phones and wireless smart meters have a direct impact on the bio-field, which is the energy field that surrounds the body that is involved with the transmission of information between cells. The frequency of these three devices is more congruent with the frequencies of our bio-field. This creates an adverse impact on the bio-field than most other devices. Therefore, the potential for a more devastating impact on our metabolism is a direct consequence. Even though we cannot eliminate our exposure to these devices, we can reduce our exposure to radiation from these devices by

1. Eliminating cordless phones from our homes or workplace.

2. Hard wire our home or office for the internet.

3. If you stay in hotels, ask for a room that is as far away from the Wi-Fi transmitter as possible.

Other electronic devices that are worth mentioning, include cell phones, laptops, television sets, alarm clocks, overhead power lines, transformers, and indoor electric wiring. Even the light bulbs we use can have adverse effects on our health—for instance, fluorescent lights, especially those with mercury vapor within them. For more information on this topic, please see the chapter in part one of my book *Heal Thyself* called "Is Modern Technology Making Us Sick?" and the chapter in part three on reducing EMF exposure.

7. Throw out your microwave oven.

We live in a "microwave society" and the allure of instantly heating food, cooking a meal or making popcorn is incredibly tempting.

It is also potentially deadly.

Microwave ovens have negative impacts on health, both through direct and indirect exposure. If you stand within four to eight feet of the microwave while it's operating, it can impact you directly, but the most common adverse effect is the impact that it has on your food and anything else heated with it and then ingested. The radiation that causes the heating effect not only goes into the food but also has detrimental impacts on biological systems when that energy is radiated back out from our food—for instance, in your intestinal track when you ingest it. It also impacts the molecular structure of certain nutrients, such as certain amino acids, and contributes to the formation of carbon-based free radicals.

The mucus membranes of the esophagus, stomach, and the small bowel are most heavily impacted by this radiation, which contributes to a number of conditions that have become very common, including increased gut permeability disorder (leaky gut syndrome), which is a major factor in the development of food sensitivities. Increased gut permeability disorder is extremely common in people with weight problems, who also often have intestinal problems like irritable bowel syndrome, constipation, gastro-esophageal reflux disease, hiatal hernias, and problems with digestion and absorption of nutrients in general.

Your microwave may not cook you, but long-term exposure and use can be harmful to your body and systems.

Exposure to Toxins through Food

Food-borne toxins are common sources of toxicity to human beings in countries like the U.S., and they contribute to metabolic dysfunction, weight gain, and difficulty losing weight. Food-borne toxins are both advertently and inadvertently added to foods. For instance, when we process foods, certain toxins are added to affect the flavor, color, or texture of food.

8. Avoid artificial sweeteners.

Artificial sweeteners have dramatic detrimental effects on our metabolism. For instance, in study after study in which researchers looked at obesity levels in people who consumed artificial sweeteners, the intake of artificial sweeteners seemed to have minimal, if any impact, on body weight. In fact, people taking in artificial sweeteners often seem to make up for the deficit in calorie intake associated with artificial sweeteners by craving other foods with actual sugar or carbohydrate calories in them. For example, people drinking artificially sweetened soft drinks often consume more pasta and other grain-based foods. There is actually a physiological reason for this because the brain and the pancreas work together to increase the release of insulin in response to the sweetener. Even when there is no actual sugar going into the system, sugar moves from the blood stream into the cells, thereby causing a type of reactive hypoglycemia that leads to even more sugar and starch cravings.

Artificial sweeteners adversely impact the body in other ways, including the acidity/alkalinity balance. Significant amounts of artificial sweeteners like aspartame, saccharin, and now maltodextran (Splenda), are extremely acidifying, which impacts metabolism negatively, and cause additional problems. For instance, aspartame is a neurotoxin and under certain circumstances, when exposed to very high temperatures, aspartame can turn into formaldehyde! This can occur when a can of soft drink is left out in the sun or is transported without proper temperature control in hot weather.

The overall long-term consequences of artificial sweeteners don't decrease problems with obesity but increase it. Artificial sweeteners create a false sense of security because we are cutting caloric intake. They are also often very addictive. For instance, when we compare those who consume diet drinks with those who consume regular soft drinks, the average consumption is actually higher for diet drinks than for regular drinks. It's not just because people feel better about the fact that they are not consuming calories, but it is also because these artificial sweeteners are specifically addicting.

The addictive potential of artificial sweeteners has become a huge problem and has even been compared to the addictive potential of certain drugs such as nicotine and even cocaine. Most people consuming artificially sweeteners can attest to that. They suffer severe withdrawal symptoms when they try to get off of these artificial sweeteners. There is an abundance of cases where severe nervous system symptoms such as tremors, feeling shaky, hypoglycemic symptoms, etc. are evident. The bottom line is, artificial sweeteners are not making us thinner: they may actually be making things worse instead.

9. Avoid foods with preservatives and other additives.

In addition to artificial sweeteners, there are other food additives that have potentially adverse impacts on metabolism. These include certain preservatives, which are made up of substances such as sulfates or nitrates. Additionally, food coloring and flavoring agents that can contribute to the toxin load in the body. Some of these chemicals can adversely impact metabolism indirectly by irritating the nervous system and stressing the body in other ways. When the body gets stressed, the nervous system gets irritated, which often leads to cravings of foods such as sugars, to counter the stressful impact. It becomes a downward spiraling cycle of "slow metabolism…gain fat…crave more sugar…slower metabolism."

In processed food there are many toxins that are not listed on the label. As a matter of fact, in America there are literally thousands of chemicals that are often included in food and don't even have to be listed on the label. In fact, the list of chemicals that do not have to be listed as ingredients or contaminants in our food or water supply exceeds a 100,000!

Some additional examples of food additives that adversely impact metabolism include partially hydrogenated fats, MSG, bromine (often added to processed grains as a preservative), aluminum (included in baking powder used in baked goods), etc.

10. Reduce exposure to pesticides, herbicides, and fungicides.

In our society we are frequently exposed to toxins literally sprayed on our food supply unless we go out of our way to reduce these exposures. These toxins include pesticides, herbicides, and fungicides. Fungicides are used in a lot of food crops we eat to reduce the growth of fungi on vegetables and fruits. Pesticides are also commonly used to reduce the negative impact of insects on crops. Herbicides are being used more often because plants have been genetically engineered to withstand the use of them, making it easier to keep crops clear of weeds. What this means is that farmers now use herbicides with impunity, meaning humans and animals are being exposed to higher and higher levels of these herbicides.

Ironically, the use of herbicides ends up weakening the plant which leads to a requirement for the use of more pesticides. This leads not to just herbicide exposure, but increased pesticide exposure for those eating genetically engineered foods. This requires more pesticides be sprayed on them, leading not just to increased herbicide exposure, but increased pesticide exposure in those eating genetically engineered foods. These herbicides and pesticides are showing up not only in our vegetables and fruits, but also in our meats and dairy products. The crops impacted by genetic engineering to make them herbicide resistant include mass cultivated crops such as corn, soy, canola, cottonseed oil, beets, cotton seed oil and all of the food products derived from those crops. In plain English, virtually all processed foods we consume have some kind of genetically engineered crop derivative in it.

Yuk.

All pesticides, herbicides, and fungicides have an adverse impact on metabolism. These toxins are fat soluble and are actually stored in our fat tissue. Fat tissue acts as a buffer against toxin overload, so when we lose weight, we release these toxins from the fat tissues back into the bloodstream. Our body must clean these out of our system through the detox organs. If they are not removed from the system, they affect the brain, nervous system, and other organs, causing us to feel ill, even as we try to do the right thing by losing weight.

The best solution is to always buy either organic or locally grown produce. This is more critical with certain foods. Logically, thin-skinned vegetables and fruits tend to be higher in pesticide concentrations because they are more easily impacted by pests and therefore, tend to be sprayed with even more pesticides, which are then drawn into the plants more readily.

All of the root vegetables tend to be more pesticide-laden, and even leafy crops like spinach and celery also are often sprayed extensively unless you specifically buy organically grown versions of these plants. Locally grown crops also tend to be sprayed less intensely even if they are not labeled organic. Many local farmers these days are using more organic growing methods but do not have the money to get their produce certified as organic. The other benefit of buying locally is you can ask the farmer himself what, if any, pesticides are used and if the produce is derived from genetically-engineered crops.

Another option that's a great solution for those who cannot afford or cannot find organic vegetables is to buy frozen organic vegetables, which tend to be more cost-effective and also more widely available and easier to purchase than fresh organic produce. It is important to note: the more people demand organic vegetables and fruits, the more they will be grown and the more competition there will be, which should decrease prices long-term.

Among vegetables and fruits, the most pesticide-ridden categories include:

- Peaches
- Nectarines
- Strawberries
- Grapes
- Apples
- Cherries
- Plums
- Potatoes

- Carrots

- Leafy vegetables

11. Minimize your intake of processed foods.

A good rule of thumb is to shop the perimeter of the grocery store instead of spending so much time in the individual aisles. Fresh products are usually kept around the perimeter, whereas processed foods will be found up and down center aisles. If something is to be found in a package on a grocery store shelf and has any significant shelf life of more than a few days, we know that something has been done to that food to give it longer shelf life. For instance, breads that are found on the shelf that you can take home and keep on your shelf for two or three weeks before they spoil contain preservatives and bad fats to protect the bread against spoilage. On the other hand, when you find bread in the refrigerator section and it is frozen, it is much more likely to be healthful. When you're focused on consuming fresh produce, you're far more likely to be healthy, have a healthy metabolism, and be able to lose weight and keep it off than if you consume a lot of processed foods.

12. Always read the labels!

Reading labels is important because at the very least, it will give you a clue of what is contained in the foods that you eat. In America, unfortunately, labels don't mean very much. There are so many bad chemicals and bad food additives that don't have to be listed on the label; it can make you sick just to discover them all. However, the label will still give you an indication of calorie count per portion, size of the portion, salt content, and the preservatives that are used. The single most important reason to read labels is to see if the food contains any artificial ingredients, artificial sweeteners, artificial preservatives, coloring agents, and flavoring agents. The simple rule is if the food contains any of those things, avoid it. Anything that has been processed by human beings is going to be toxic to your health in some way, shape, or form, so your best bet is to avoid these altogether whenever possible.

There are exceptions to the rule, of course. In time of crisis, any food is better than none, and under those circumstances, food preservation becomes essential. There are certain dehydration processes that give you the best opportunity to maintain nutritional quality while minimizing the use of preservatives. Consider stocking up on some of these items if you are concerned about a possible crisis down the line—for example, if you live in areas prone to weather-related disasters.

13. Limit the intake of toxic drugs and supplements.

By definition, every drug and pharmaceutical is a toxin. With the exception of a small minority of drugs that are actual replicas of the body's own chemicals, (such as the hormones estradiol, testosterone, and cortisol) the vast majority of drugs are artificial and contribute to organ stress on the kidneys, liver, and other organs focused on detoxification.

Any pharmaceutical can have a negative impact on metabolism, directly or indirectly. Whenever possible, target the source of the illness rather than try to eliminate symptoms.

Over-the-counter drugs

The use of over-the-counter drugs, which are used with impunity by the vast majority of our population, are used with very little thought as to the adverse impact that these drugs can have on health and well-being. What makes this tragic is the false security these drugs have and how they impact not only our adult population, but our children.

Commonly used drugs, such as painkillers containing acetaminophen, can have adverse effects on liver and kidney function. Drugs such as non-steroidal anti-inflammatories (like ibuprofen) can adversely impact kidneys and intestinal tract lining which tends to accelerate the wear and tear on joints, muscles, and tendons. This further impacts on our ability to lose weight and maintain a healthy metabolism.

It is also important to remember that a large proportion of vitamins and minerals on the market are toxic in some way. They may not always contain toxins, but the manner in which they are produced and what they are made from can create a level of toxicity. It has been estimated that upwards of 80% of the supplements on the market are not health promoting but may actually be disease promoting because of the nutrient source. For instance, the vast majority of multi-vitamins have one or more ingredient in them from potentially toxic sources, such as from GMO corn or GMO soy. Vitamin C almost always comes from genetically engineered corn (GMO corn). Vitamin E (d-alpha-tocopherol) almost always comes from genetically engineered soy (GMO soy), and d-l-alpha-tocopherol is synthetic vitamin E and is even more harmful.

Even when we try to do what we think is healthy, we can end up doing more harm than good if we don't educate ourselves.

Beware of the Air You Breathe

Indoor air quality is as important, if not more important, than outdoor air quality because we spend so much time indoors. Indoor air pollution is an issue that most people don't understand. Indoor air pollutants come from many different sources including wall-to-wall carpets, furniture, drywall, paint, and household chemicals. The chemicals and toxins we are exposed to indoors are too numerous to list, but include chemicals such as formaldehyde, a variety of different household cleaners, pesticides and dust mite excrement. These affect indoor air quality and can cause allergic reactions and in some cases can literally poison the body.

Also worth mentioning are micro-related toxins, including fungal spores, molds, and dust mites' excrement that also get into the air ducts and air condition systems of our homes and businesses. Mold is often found in buildings that have sustained water damage. The mold is not always visible, especially in the walls and the floors that have been affected by water. If not properly dried out and decontaminated, the mold remains, even after a coat of paint. Any building that has water damage in the walls and the floors will also have a much higher likelihood of mold overgrowth and can lead to black mold exposure, which can adversely affect our health.

14. Use air purifiers in your home.

Consider the use of air purifiers in your home, especially in the rooms where you spend a lot of time. There are also systems that can be put in place in the air conditioning systems of homes or offices to clean up the air. HEPA filters can be used in the air conditioning systems or a separate unit with HEPA filters can be used to filter out small particular pollutants from the air by room. Vacuum cleaners with HEPA filters are becoming more commonplace, which makes it easier to clean the indoor environments and carpets. With a HEPA filter, the dust and toxins are actually removed instead of recirculating them as happens with bag vacuum cleaners.

15. Add some live plants to your décor.

There are natural ways to improve indoor air quality, include the use of indoor plants around your home and business. You may consider adding full-spectrum light bulbs to help keep these plants strong and vibrant. Another option is to place the plants close to the windows where the sun shines through for at least a small part of the day. These plants not only improve the air quality, they provide a warm and pleasant environment.

16. Minimize indoor air pollutants.

There are a number of things we can do to reduce the number of air pollutants indoors. For example, if you own animals, be sure to clean animal dander from rugs and carpets thoroughly on a regular basis. The most allergenic type of animal dander tends to be from cats. Another indoor pollutant that must be minimized are dust mites. Many people are sensitive to dust mite excrement and the most common source for this type of exposure is the mattress and the pillows we sleep on. It is important to use pillow covers and mattress covers that are dust-mite-resistant. Carpets also harbor dust mites and in some instances in order to remove them, the carpets have to be treated or removed completely.

Brandy Lucas has lost over 50 pounds since she started working for us. She has seen major improvements in overall health and emotional well-being.

###

I learned to hate elevators.

Becoming healthy and losing the extra fat was so easy, I don't know why I didn't do it sooner. The simple logic of Dr. De Wet's advice (using the stairs instead of the elevator) was so simple, yet as a habit—transformative.

I lost about 40 pounds in all over about four months. While I wasn't dealing with any other health problems at the time, I still felt that it was important to lose weight. I feel now like a huge amount of stress has been lifted off of me. I have the stamina to endure longer periods of exercise, and I don't get tired while playing with my children. I am so much happier now, and my mood has changed drastically.

By following Dr. De Wet's guidelines, I have been able to maintain my weight fairly easily. Losing weight before was a very difficult task, and when I did lose it, I would gain it back very quickly. What I especially loved about Dr. De Wet's practice was the fact that he shows a 100 percent commitment to the well-being of his patients, to help them on all fronts, including the emotional roots of their health challenges, and not just by treating symptoms. In fact, what makes him so remarkable is the fact that Dr. De Wet has used the same techniques on himself and has shown how well it works through his own experience. I love the idea of following someone's recommendations after they have shown it to be successful and helpful in their own experience. It makes everything much more real.

Dr. De Wet used the β HCG weight loss program to help me lose weight, but I also really felt that his knowledge and understanding played a vital role in my ability to lose weight. Every time I would talk to him, I would walk away feeling so much better about myself and where I was going with my life. I no longer feel like I have to be obese. I know now I have another choice, and Dr. De Wet gave me that. I look forward to reaching my goal weight and just being overall healthy so that I can watch my children grow up and participate in their lives fully.

The biggest challenge I faced as I lost my weight was the emotional factor. I faced many bumps (emotional) along the way, and it was very difficult to deal with them, but I had to deal with them in order to be able to lose my weight and keep it off.

My entire lifestyle has changed now because I don't stress about food any longer. I've learned what is good for my body and what isn't, so it makes it that much easier to know what to eat. I really feel like I now have the knowledge I need to live a healthy lifestyle, so I can continue to lose weight until I reach my optimal weight and then be able to maintain that weight.

Chapter Six:
Lifestyle: Time to Release the Fat and MOVE

"When you eat one or two meals per day, you are much more likely to GAIN weight than if you eat five or six meals per day."

—Dr. Pieter De Wet

The physiology of the body is influenced by everything we do—every habit we have and everything we do on a daily basis. Of course diet and exercise play major roles, but so do sleep habits, how we deal with stress, water intake, and how well we maintain our alkalinity-acidity balance.

The Benefits of Optimal Sleep

A number of studies have shown that people who do not get enough sleep have more problems with obesity than those who do. There is a direct correlation between sleep deprivation and the slow metabolism. Lack of sleep also contributes to abnormal or dysfunctional eating habits.

The average adult should get somewhere between seven to nine hours of sleep per night, although the amount of sleep needed varies from person to person. Children need even more sleep than adults. The younger you are, the more sleep you need. Seniors often have lower sleep requirements than younger adults. (Yet many seniors tend to complain more about insomnia!) Sleep deprivation is a relatively common problem in our society and is one of the reasons many people have to eat more in order to try to keep their energy levels up. This, of course, adds to the obesity spiral. With an increase of food intake comes an increased chance of obesity and sleep apnea which leads to poor sleep quality. With poor sleep quality comes increased fatigue and then…you get the idea. It spirals down from there.

When we are sleep deprived, we also tend to make poorer choices in terms of *what* we eat. Additionally, there are certain dietary factors that contribute to sleep deprivation. People often revert to consuming more calories in order to get their energy going. The increased caloric intake often involves food that has an adverse impact on the hormones. Sugars and starches are the worst culprits for affecting the hormones which control our metabolism.

There is a direct correlation between the stimulants that people consume and increased body weight. A lot of people literally stay on stimulants constantly in order to function. It's a little bit like taking speed. These same people cannot sleep at night because they're so wound up with all the stimulants in their systems. Other chemicals like artificial sweeteners also contribute to poor sleep because they act as stimulants and irritants to the system.

Another reason sleep deprivation is common is the fact that we live in a society where high stress levels are so prevalent they have become the norm. We live in a much more advanced society than our ancestors, and have so much more on our minds. With so many decision points to resolve, it naturally creates overwhelm and stress. Additionally, vast chunks of our society have jobs that force people to work unusual hours. For example, many professionals have to work the night shift, this contributes to an individuals' sleep deprivation.

Other contributing factors to sleep deprivation include:

1. Watching television and working on a computer right before bedtime. Doing those things within two hours of going to bed activates increased beta brain wave activity, which means that these activities stimulate the brain instead of helping us relax towards sleep.

2. Exposure to electromagnetic fields on a chronic basis, including in our bedrooms, also contributes to sleeplessness. This includes exposure to Wi-Fi, an alarm clock that sits too close to your body when you're asleep, and the cordless phone that is often right next to the bed on a base that radiates EMF. These devices all cause considerable interference with the body's own bio field, thereby disrupting the communication between cells. This is especially

true of Wi-Fi systems, cordless phones, and wireless smart meters installed on our homes and businesses by utility companies.

There are a number of hormones that are affected by sleep deprivation and excessive stress. Melatonin is one of them, and adequate melatonin production happens to be critical for healthful sleep. When you are sleep deprived, your pineal gland does not make enough melatonin, and this causes you to become more stress-vulnerable. Adequate melatonin production is critical for optimal hormonal production cycles, such as the circadian rhythm (adrenal hormonal production cycle). It is critical to maintain normal hormonal cycles in the body for optimal metabolism. Melatonin is also the most important antioxidant that your body needs and is by far the most powerful one created. When you lose melatonin production, your body is more vulnerable to oxidation stress, which is associated with the burning of oxygen and the creation of oxygen free radicals that are normally buffered by antioxidants such as melatonin. When you don't have enough antioxidants in your body, that leads to more inflammation in your body, including inflammation associated with obesity (remember, obesity is by definition an inflammatory state). This is a slippery slope towards gaining more and more weight.

There are other hormones that impact sleep deprivation. When you are sleep deprived, your adrenal glands are forced to go into overdrive and tend to make more cortisone, which is the most prominent stress-related hormone produced when there is chronic or ongoing stress.

Acute stress, on the other hand, is associated with the release of epinephrine, also called adrenaline, which does not have the kind of long-term negative effects on metabolism that cortisone has. The body can handle short bursts of stress at times, but it is chronic stress that makes us sick, fat and tired. One of the ways that excessive cortisone levels impacts our ability to burn calories is it causes a slowdown in our metabolism and an increased tendency to store calories in the form of long-chained sugars and fat (glucagon and lipids).

When you are sleep deprived, you disrupt the manufacturing of dopamine in the brain. This is the neurotransmitter that is associated with joy, and sleep deprived people tend to have less of the "joy" factor than those who are well rested. Serotonin is a neurotransmitter that is associated with sleep and mood control. In other words, it is our brain's natural antidepressant. 5-hydroxytryptophan and tryptophan are precursors to serotonin, and a deficiency in either of these amino acids or sleep deprivation can lead to a reduced production of serotonin. This leads to negative consequences, including increased propensity towards depression and anxiety. Conversely, when you get enough sleep, your adrenals tend to function better and cortisone levels tend to be lower, which helps the brain to make adequate amounts of dopamine and serotonin. This promotes a healthy metabolism and healthy body weight.

People who do not get a full eight hours of sleep seem to do fine if they get adequate naps during other times of the day. There are many type A personalities—people who thrive on less nighttime sleep—who take daytime naps and are able to function at a very high level with healthy metabolisms. Even if you get adequate rest at night, there seems to be a benefit to short naps, especially in the early afternoon, right after lunch. Sleep deprived people are much less willing to exercise, so sleep has a direct effect on your attitude toward exercise and physical activity.

Nutrition Myths, Facts, and Solutions: The Best Diet

Everyone knows that obesity and diet are directly related, but it is important to understand that there is no perfect diet for everyone. Every human being is different, and we have to take these differences into account when we design the ideal diet that is most likely to promote optimal health, metabolism and well-being. There is a glut of books written about all kinds of different diets, and they all seem to disagree with each other and insist that *their* protocol or program is the best. There is the Atkins Diet; the South Beach Diet; the High-Fat, Low-Carb Diet; the Low Fat, High Carb Diet; etc. There are a few people who do well on these diets, but most people will fail over time. They may discover that one particular diet works well for a while, but then they start responding negatively to that diet.

For example, the Atkins Diet works very well for many people in the beginning, but after a while, it can contribute to certain health problems such as gall bladder problems. This is especially true if that person is following a very high protein diet focusing mainly on animal proteins. A high protein diet can be very stressful on the kidneys. This is because of the high concentration of protein breakdown products (the chemicals that are created by the body when it breaks down proteins) that have to be excreted through the kidneys. This puts excessive stress on the kidneys. Before you start on a diet, it is important to determine your unique characteristics so that you can choose the diet that will work best for you.

At the Quantum Healing Institute, www.qhiwellness.com, we treat every person as an individual. No two people are alike. An extremely thorough history and analysis is our normal protocol. In order to design the best diet for someone, we look at these key factors:

1. **Blood Type**

There is a link between blood types and metabolic types. People who are Type O blood types generally do well eating diets higher in protein—including red meat, veal, lamb, and duck—turkey and chicken are less optimal for Type O's but acceptable on occasion, with pork being more counterproductive. Most Type O's tolerate some forms of seafood, although they don't usually do well with shellfish and also have a tendency to have problems with freshwater fish. Most non-starchy vegetables are good options for Type O's, but the starchy vegetables like potatoes and possibly sweet potatoes may also cause problems. They also tend to do well on most fruits except the higher glycemic index fruits, especially oranges, cantaloupe, and honeydew. They don't do well with grains, especially corn and wheat. Beans are generally good but many Type O's don't do very well on some of the higher glycemic index beans like kidney beans and black-eyed peas. They also don't do well with other carbohydrates that are on the high end of the glycemic index and most dairy products. Simple sugars are also a problem, but nuts and seeds work well for them (except for peanuts and cashews). Most Type O's also do relatively well eating less often and are more tolerant to eating once or twice a day in contrast to an A blood type. A Type O is much more likely to be tolerant to eating once or twice a day rather than a person with Type A blood.

For Type O's, the ideal diet would include a main meal that consists of a serving of meat—ideally from an organic source—if the person is not a vegetarian. Fish, including red snapper, orange roughy, or wild salmon, may also be good up to a couple of times a week. They should combine a serving of meat with a portion of non-starchy vegetables. If a grain is consumed as part of a meal, the lower glycemic index grains tend to be the best, including quinoa, amaranth, buckwheat and kamut. Rice is not great for Type O's either, but wild rice and brown rice can be good options.

Blood Type A's, on the other hand, are usually on the opposite side of the spectrum compared to Type O's. They tend to be carbohydrate or mixed metabolic types and they may have problems making a sufficient amount of acids or enzymes, especially to digest heavier animal proteins such as red meat. They are more likely to have vitamin B12 deficiencies because of this digestive issue and are also more likely to have problems like chronic fatigue, autoimmune diseases, hypothyroidism, and immune dysfunction, resulting in greater vulnerability towards infections. Type A's tend to make great vegetarians. The modified fast listed later in this chapter is an absolutely fantastic diet for this blood type. Type A's, in other words, do well when they de-emphasize meats and when the meats they do eat are lighter meats like chicken or turkey.

For those Type A's who choose not to be vegetarians, they tend to do well on most types of fish and meats from smaller animals: rabbit, quail, and so forth, as well as pork and turkey. Dairy, eggs, and whole grains are usually good choices for Type A's unless they are gluten-sensitive, which seems to be happening more and more in all blood types. Type A's also do well with beans and vegetables of all types, except bell peppers, tomatoes, cabbage, potatoes, and sweet potatoes. They do well on most fruits, except for some tropical fruits like bananas, oranges, mangos, and papaya. They do well on most nuts and seeds, including peanuts and cashews. Type A's tend to do better eating smaller, more frequent meals.

Blood types B and AB tend to do best on modern diets and as far as metabolic typing, would be more likely to be carbohydrate or carbohydrate-protein (mixed) types. People of both blood type B and AB tend to make great vegetarians because they have difficulties with most types of animal flesh except for fish. Like Type A's, AB's do well on most shellfish. Most poultry, except for turkey, is problematic for them, as is pork. Dairy and eggs are often beneficial, as are grains like oats, rice, millet, and spelt. Once again, wheat and corn present a problem because of the increasing incidence of sensitivity to GMO corn and gluten containing grains. They also tend to have problems with certain nuts, including peanuts, cashews, and pistachios. They do well with most types of beans, vegetables, and fruits.

You can find more information on eating for your blood type in Dr. Peter J. D'Adamo's book *Eat Right for Your Type*.

2. **Metabolic Type**

There is some correlation between metabolic type and blood type. For example, more Type O's tend to be protein types, but there are frequent exceptions to this rule. The same applies to Type A's, who tend to be carbohydrate types or mixed types. As far as metabolic type goes, you can be one of three types. You can be a protein type, a carbohydrate type, or a mixed type. Those who are protein types tend to do better on fewer meals per day (1 or 2 meals per day). However, if fewer meals are consumed, they have to be earlier in the day rather than later in the day. Even though protein types can tolerate one meal a day rather well, it is not ideal to do so because it slows down metabolism. Carbohydrate types, on the other hand, do much better when they consume smaller and more frequent meals (4 to 6 meals per day). Carbohydrate types tend to do poorly when they eat fewer times and tend to be prone to reactive hypoglycemic episodes. Mixed metabolic types tend to find themselves somewhere in the middle between these two extremes. They do better with more frequent meals (3 to 4 meals per day) and also tend to be a little bit more resilient to skipping meals than carbohydrate types.

In order to figure out what your metabolic type is, we look at your response to certain types of foods and certain eating patterns. We look at your hunger patterns, energy patterns, and mental well-being patterns in response to the intake of certain food types and certain eating patterns to try to identify what your metabolic type is. If someone does better on a diet that is heavy in proteins as far as mental alertness or energy, then we know that they are probably a protein type. If they are also able to go for a long time between meals without eating, then they are more likely to be a protein type. On the other hand, carbohydrate types are characterized by the fact that they tend to do better mentally and energy-wise when they eat more frequent meals and when they eat meals with more carbohydrate type foods, whereas they do not do well at all with long spaces between meals.

3. Food Sensitivities

The majority of the population has some degree of food sensitivities. With genetic engineering of foods, microwaving, and an increased incidence of leaky gut syndrome (increased gut permeability disorder), food sensitivities are spiraling out of control. Symptoms of food sensitivity can run the gamut from irritable bowel syndrome, acid reflux disease, constipation, and diarrhea to hypoglycemia, gall bladder problems, or appendicitis. Other disorders involving food sensitivities can include inflammatory bowel disease, fibromyalgia, irritable bladder, chronic fatigue, and any kind of pain syndromes—joints, muscles, or otherwise. Even asthma, eczema, sinus allergies, and angina can be aggravated by food sensitivities.

Here are the most common food sensitivities:

Cow dairy	Black pepper	Pork
Gluten (Wheat, barley, kamut, rye spelt and oats, etc.)	Food additives	Tomatoes
	Artificial sweeteners	Strawberries
		Bananas
	Preservatives	Apples
	Carrying agents	Almonds
Corn		Walnuts
Soy	Mustard	Baker's yeast
Eggs	Coffee	Brewer's yeast
Cane sugar	White potatoes	Beets
Peanuts		
Shellfish	Beef	
Oranges	Chicken	

There are numerous ways to identify food sensitivities, including blood testing, skin testing, and bio-energetic testing. There is even a clinical test that can be done, which is to check your pulse rate 30 minutes to an hour after you eat. If your pulse rate rises by at least 15 beats per minute or more after you eat your food and stays up for more than 30 minutes compared to your base pulse rate, it is almost certain that it is a response to a food sensitivity, which was triggered by the meal in which that food was eaten.

A major reason we are seeing increasing numbers of people with food sensitivities is because of the genetic engineering of foods. This phenomenon of food production is affecting nearly all food categories. The biggest culprits include corn, soy, canola, cottonseed, rapeseed, and beets. Even supplements and vitamins made from these genetically-engineered sources, such as Vitamin E and Vitamin C are causing problems.

4.   Overall alkalinity or acidity balance

The level of alkalinity or acidity in your body is vital to know when determining your ideal diet. Most people with obesity and other chronic illnesses tend to be acidic and do much better when they properly alkalinize their bodies. When we consume more fresh vegetables and fruits and less animal protein, starch, sugar, and grains, we alkalinize more readily and heal more easily from these pathologies.

5.   Overall level of health and specific health challenges

When people are in relatively poor health, there are specific consequences. For instance, when someone is in generally poor health, they tend to have digestive tracts that do not function properly. A person in poor health tends to have a higher incidence of leaky gut syndrome. This, of course, needs to be repaired for better digestion and the assimilation of nutrients. To repair the gut lining, we can supplement with licorice root extract, aloe vera, and the amino acid L-glutamine. In these same individuals, supplementation with digestive enzymes and digestive acids may be needed in order to improve digestion and assimilation.

Other health challenges that impact what a healthy diet would look like for an individual include;

- Dental challenges

- Intestinal diseases
- Pancreatic pathologies
- Gallbladder problems
- And scores of other maladies

For someone with poor oral health, this may impact their ability to chew. Obviously, the need to pulverize their food before it is swallowed is necessary. It must be mixed with saliva before they swallow it in order to get the digestive process going in the mouth itself. Other conditions that can impact the ability to digest include gallbladder disease. There is a notable increase in people who are having their gallbladders removed. When the gall bladder is removed, it may be difficult for those individuals to digest fats and they may need supplementation to restore this ability to digest. These supplements may include ox bile and certain enzymes–both of which assist in the proper digestion and the absorption of fats.

6. Overall level of toxicity

When it comes to metabolism, overall toxicity levels are important. On a physical level, the more toxicity in our bodies, the greater the negative impact will be on our metabolism and ability to lose weight. It also means the more toxic you are, the more careful you should be about what you ingest. We want to minimize the load of additional toxicity that we accumulate through the consumption of foods with toxic additives. On the other hand, it's also a good idea when there is a lot of toxicity, to do what we can to support our detox mechanisms and detox organs. Please visit www.qhiwellness.com for information on my recommendation for detox support.

7. Availability and affordability of healthy promoting foods

A lot of people who live in certain parts of the country and some parts of the world do not have many organic food choices. In fact, in some parts of the world, fresh produce of any kind is hard to find. This includes the inner cities of America. When organic vegetables and fruits are not available, good options include the thicker skinned vegetables and fruits. Thicker skinned vegetables tend to be good options, even if you don't have organic vegetables available. Washing your foods with water and hydrogen peroxide or acidic water from a water ionizer is a great way to get rid of the surface toxins on produce. Frozen organic vegetables are also an option and may be easier to obtain than fresh organic produce.

8. Social situation

In order to be successful with any lifestyle change, it is incredibly important to work with your social environment. Without a support system of those around you, setbacks and failure become commonplace. A dysfunctional social environment can lead to self-sabotage both directly and indirectly. It is critical for us to communicate to others how they can support us in our efforts to be healthier and in return, for us to support them with their same goals. If you are unable to remove yourself from toxic relationships on a long-term basis, seek out and nurture positive, encouraging friends and family who share the same empowering beliefs you have and are developing.

9. Belief systems related to nutrition

Some people have dysfunctional belief systems when it comes to nutrition. Many believe they can eat anything and be healthy. That's not a very healthy belief system to have, and these people usually end up with very serious health problems. They often end up with the "see doctor too often" consequence. Unfortunately, a lot of people are closed to the idea that their food choices have huge impacts on their overall health and well-being.

The first thing you need to do about your diet is to go through the checklist discussed and figure out what your ideal diet should look like in order to tackle metabolic problems successfully. Eating perfectly may not be critical if you are in great health and only a little bit overweight. On the other hand, if you are even slightly overweight and have associated health problems such as diabetes, hypertension, and so forth, then you may want and need to shed that extra weight. Even if you are not obese or overweight, you may have an increased risk of developing diabetes or hypertension. Consider losing 10 to 15 pounds in order to attain your optimal body weight and clear or reduce your predisposition to the disease. Your optimal body weight may put you in the lower range of normal in terms of body mass index based on your body frame. Remember, body mass index is just one indicator. It is not the only measurement of optimal health and weight. Look at waist measurements, body frame, and overall health status to define what your ideal body weight would be in order to optimize your chances to resolve any chronic health problems.

Vitality Rating of Food

When figuring out what kinds of foods to eat, we should be aware of the vitality rating of the foods that we consume. The vitality rating has to do with the 'aliveness' of food. It has actual life energy—not just calories. For instance, if you eat a hamburger, you will find that the vitality rating is very low. The cattle are no longer alive, of course. It has been processed, refrigerated and cooked. Both the meat and the bread tend to have a low vitality rating. It is close to what is called, "dead foods." If you add some fresh vegetables to the hamburger, that will increase the vitality rating. On the other hand, when you consume fresh vegetables grown organically in your own backyard, it will have a very high vitality rating. The vegetables are still alive. Live foods are more likely to contribute to better health and well-being. Moreover, live foods will make it easier to lose excess fat than consuming a low vitality, dead hamburger.

The vitality rating of organic fruits and vegetables is higher than the vitality ratings of regularly grown fruits and vegetables that has been sitting on a store shelf for days or weeks. Fruits, for example, on store shelves are often picked green and ripened through artificial means just before they are placed on the shelves. This causes them to have a much lower vitality rating and nutrient density than organically-grown fruits that are picked ripe and then consumed relatively quickly after harvest.

Another way to frame vitality rating is to think of it as light in solid form. The foods that we consume are products of the sun acting on life forms such as plants. Plants make oxygen and consume carbon from carbon dioxide which is the main building block the plants we consume. Animals, in turn, eat these plants and turn them into flesh that we eat. When we're talking about vitality rating, we are literally talking about the light content of food. The fresher and more organic the food is, the higher the 'light' content of the food and the higher the vitality rating.

Foods that are cooked at high temperatures have their vitality ratings markedly reduced and making them potentially more detrimental to health. Even meat loses its vitality rating when overcooked. This is why eating rare meat is healthier than overcooked or grilled meat that has been charred on the outside. The charring of meat actually creates more toxicity that is harmful to the intestinal tract and can increase the risk of intestinal tract malignancies.

A word of caution: ground meat should always be cooked more thoroughly to prevent ingesting dangerous E. coli and other pathogenic bacteria.

Basic Principles for Healthful Eating

When I see someone with dysfunctional metabolism, anyone with a chronic illness, or even those who just want to do a proper detox protocol, I recommend they start with a modified fast, which is phase one of my *Green Life Diet*.

Green Life Diet

I started using the *Green Life Diet* with my patients in 1994, and I've treated over 10,000 patients with this diet with great success. The *Green Life Diet* is a set of standard recommendations for eating that is congruent other dietary recommendations that have been popularized in other books. The reason why I've had great success with my *Green Life Diet* over the years is not solely due to the soundness of the dietary recommendations in it, but because I have combined it with certain behavior modification strategies. These strategies include the rooting out of dysfunctional belief systems and helping people to accept more empowering belief systems about what is healthy and what is not. What also made my program unique is the fact that we track down the emotional roots of dysfunctional eating habits. We are also successful at helping people get rid of self-defeating behaviors, including dysfunctional eating habits.

Recall Healing forms the lynchpin of this approach. What also makes our approach to healthy eating unique is the fact that we teach people to individualize effectively based on their uniquenesses, including their metabolic type, blood type, food sensitivities, and so forth. In other words, the basic principle here is that there is no one perfect diet that works for every single human being on this planet.

The Green Life Diet is primarily based on the concept of glycemic index, which is used as the primary framework for the four phases of the diet, including the Modified Fast. The Modified Fast is a very strict, and for most, temporarily a very low glycemic index dietary phase. The Modified Fast is very helpful for those who want to be very aggressive in the detoxification process, including those who are very ill. It will also assist those dealing with very severe insulin resistance and those who have severely dysfunctional metabolisms. Phase one of the *Green Life Diet* is a little bit more expansive than the Modified Fast because it adds a few organic animal products into the mix. Phase two expands that list further to include some moderate glycemic index foods. Phase three adds in a few higher glycemic index foods like whole grains but still avoid the bad foods that we typically consume, such as highly processed foods.

The Modified Fast is usually recommended for two to six weeks and helpful in alkalinizing the body, improving immune system function, decreasing inflammation, and decreasing yeast overgrowth. The Modified Fast is a great launch pad for losing quite a few pounds right off the bat. It is not uncommon for those on the Modified Fast to lose two to three pounds per week. Many people feel energized when on the Modified Fast, although some may feel drained because of the acceleration of detoxification that naturally occurs. Also, those who are blood type O or protein metabolic types may feel somewhat drained during the Modified Fast. The critical key here is to eat more frequently (4 to 6 times per day) when following the Modified Fast. If you get too drained while on the Modified Fast, this would be a good reason to move right to phase one of the *Green Life Diet*.

The Modified Fast includes the following low glycemic index vegetables:

Artichokes   Asparagus

Brussel sprouts	Cauliflower	Bell peppers
	Celery	Spinach
String beans	Cucumbers	Squash
Green beans	Eggplant	Tomatoes
Bean sprouts	Lettuce	Turnips
Bamboo shoots	Onions	Water chestnuts
Broccoli	Kale	Watercress
Cabbage	Parsley	Zucchini
	Pea pods	

It also includes the following list of low glycemic index fruits:

Avocados	Plums	Blackberries
Fresh cranberries	Strawberries	Boysenberries
	Blueberries	Cantaloupe
Cherries	Raspberries	Lemons
Grapefruit	Kiwis	Limes

Fresh fruits are always best, although frozen fruits can be used instead if fresh is hard to find. Snacks between meals should be made up of nuts or seeds. In some cases,

175

powdered medical food used to make shakes or smoothies can be used to supplement the diet, although it is very important that they do not contain any artificial sweeteners, toxic ingredients such as GMO corn or GMO soy, or non-organic dairy. Rice protein is hypoallergenic and tends to be health promoting. Organic whey can be very healthful as a primary ingredient in these medical foods. Visit www.qhiwellness.com for a list of powdered medical foods.

Cooked dry beans and lentils are also good options, although these should be taken in small amounts by people who are suffering from insulin resistance (Those with more severe obesity, hypertension, diabetes, hyperlipidemia). Super green foods such as chlorella, spirulina and barley greens can be added and are perfect for patients who are trying to detoxify and alkalinize their bodies.

Healthy fats like extra virgin olive oil, extra virgin coconut oil, grape seed oil, sesame oil, and flax oil should also be included with this diet. It is very important that you avoid foods you are sensitive to while you're on the Modified Fast. You may have to do some work to find out which foods you are sensitive to by eliminating them from your diet one at a time if you seem to be having adverse reactions to the Modified Fast.

Phase One of the *Green Life Diet*

Phase One includes all of the foods listed under Modified Fast, plus a few additions. Most vegetables are part of Phase One except for starchy vegetables like potatoes and sweet potatoes. Certain vegetables like cauliflower, carrots, and beets can be included in Phase One but should be eaten in moderation only, especially if they are consumed in juice form. Fruits listed under Phase One of the *Green Life Diet* are exactly the same as those listed under the Modified Fast. By the way, dried fruits are probably not a good option in either of these phases because dried fruits tend to have higher glycemic indexes than the fresh versions of the same fruits.

Most nuts are good in either the Modified Fast or phase one, except for the higher glycemic index nuts, including peanuts, cashews, pistachios, and macadamia nuts. However, we should keep in mind not to consume too many nuts and seeds because they are rather dense in terms of calorie content. Also make sure that the nuts you do eat are fresh. Rancid nuts contain rancid oils, and fungi associated with them that can be toxic to your body. You can usually smell when nuts are going bad.

Phase one of the Green Life Diet includes meats and eggs, and depending on your health and blood type, organic dairy may also be included. All animal proteins should be organic (or grass-fed, in the case of red meat). Again, these recommendations would be modified to some degree, depending on your blood type.

Lean beef	Rabbit	Duck
Buffalo	Venison	Ostrich
Lamb	Turkey	Emu
Veal	Chicken	Goose

Fresh ocean fish is a good option for Phase One, although freshwater fish should be limited, especially bottom-dwelling fish, like catfish. Be careful of shellfish. Pollution of the oceans has become a serious concern in certain areas where shellfish are harvested. Eggs can be included in phase one as long as they are organic and soft poached or soft boiled. It is important to note that the Modified Fast and the *Green Life Diet* Phase One help to normalize the body's insulin response and therefore can be helpful and even curative in numerous diseases that are based on insulin resistance, which have been mentioned previously.

The *Green Life Diet* phase two foods includes some moderate glycemic index foods and all foods included under the Modified Fast and Green Life Diet phase one. Patients who have responded well to the first two phases (modified fast and phase one) of the *Green Life Diet* who are in good health and at a relatively healthy body weight are ready to move into phase two. Even patients with mild weight issues, controlled hypertension or even mild diabetes can move into phase two.

In Phase Two, you are allowed to add in certain additional vegetables in, such as:

Sweet potato	Tomato puree	Jerusalem artichoke
Winter squash	Rutabaga	Red potatoes

It's also important to realize that white potatoes can be included in this phase, but it depends on how they are cooked. For example, baked or scalloped white potatoes are in the medium glycemic index, but mashed potatoes are high glycemic index. Of course, French fries, fried in oil should always be avoided because they are processed and entirely unhealthy. Also keep lima beans, black-eyed peas, and kidney beans to smaller amounts during this phase.

Some further additions include moderate glycemic index grains like:

- Buckwheat
- Wild rice
- Corn-on-the-cob
- Quinoa
- Brown rice
- Slow cooked Steel-cut oatmeal

Limited amounts of other whole grains can be included in phase two, such as:

- Steel-cut oats
- Barley
- Millet
- Spelt
- Buckwheat
- Kamut
- Quinoa
- Amaranth
- Rye
- Non-GMO corn & wheat
- Brown & wild rice
- Whole grain crackers

Additions in the fruit category for phase two include:

- Apricots
- Peaches
- Nectarines
- Blueberries
- Boysenberries
- Pineapples
- Bananas
- Cantaloupes
- Honeydew
- Apples
- Pears
- Grapes
- Kiwi

Some of these fruits are actually higher glycemic index fruits, but these contain natural sugars, which do not usually pose as much of a problem to our metabolism. They are generally appropriate to eat during this phase of the diet. People who are in phase two should avoid processed grains and simple sugars. Tropical fruits such as oranges and mangos can be consumed during this phase but should be consumed in limited amounts.

Phase Three takes all of the foods that are included in the first two phases and adds all foods back in, but in very specific forms. Processed grains and packaged foods should be avoided during all phases of the *Green Life Diet*. In phase three, unrestricted access to whole grains is allowed (including wheat and corn) and all types of vegetables, beans, nuts and seeds.

Food Combining Rules

Within the *Green Life Diet*, there are certain rules that should be followed as you combine different foods. If these rules are not followed, certain adverse effects can occur, even when consuming an otherwise healthful diet.

1. Eat fruits alone. Fruit should be eaten for breakfast or snacks at least 30 minutes before a meal or more than two hours after a meal. Fruits and vegetables can be eaten together because they are digested at a relatively higher Ph than proteins. In order to digest proteins effectively, a higher stomach acid level is needed. When you combine fruits and higher glycemic index vegetables, with, for example, animal protein you often slow down digestion, which leads to fermentation. Lower glycemic vegetables, on the other hand, are fine to combine with proteins in the

stomach. This should exclude starchy vegetables, which tend to interfere with the digestion of high protein foods.

2. Don't eat fruit with cereal. If you eat fruit with a starch, then you're increasing the absorption of sugar, so you get an increased insulin response when dealing with hyperinsulinemia or insulin resistance.

3. Eat grains and starchy vegetables with lower glycemic index vegetables. If you are going to eat grains, eat them with vegetables but not with high-protein foods like meats for the same reasons as described in number one.

4. Avoid eating animal proteins within three hours of starches. Combining animal proteins with starches delays stomach emptying and contributes to the development of conditions such as reflux, constipation and makes it harder to maintain a healthy metabolism.

5. If you're Type A or Type AB, you probably should avoid red meats or pork, especially at lunch or dinner. If you are Type O or Type B, (especially if you have more of a protein metabolism) you will do better and might prefer animal proteins such as red meat or pork.

6. If you haven't figured out your metabolic type or your blood type yet, then opt for fish, chicken, or turkey to get your animal proteins. These represent lighter animal proteins that are easier to digest. Red meat and pork are hard to digest for some people, especially Type A's and maybe Type AB's to some degree.

7. Do not eat any foods more often than every three to four days to reduce the likelihood of developing food sensitivities. Most people in our society are suffering from

food sensitivities. Sensitivities contribute to metabolism problems and other digestive diseases. It is also more likely that someone with food sensitivities will have problems with cravings and food addictions. This makes it harder to achieve success with rehabilitation of metabolism.

Sometimes supplementation is necessary to provide the proper nutrients needed in a diet, although supplements also have a downside because they tend to have lower vitality ratings unless they are part of a super green or multi-herbal combination. Nutrients extracted from their original vital source and put into a capsule basically lose their vital essence.

Whenever you are trying to put together a healthy eating plan to combat your metabolic dysfunction and your weight problems, it is important and helpful to understand there are certain critical nutrients that will help you in this quest. These may include:

- Chromium and vanadium, which help to normalize sugar metabolism
- Magnesium will help regulate insulin sensitivity and muscle function
- Iodine, which is critical for thyroid function and normal metabolism

Thirteen Diet Myths to Resolve

There are dozens of myths circulating through our population about dieting that need to be debunked if we want to be successful with weight loss and getting healthy. We will discuss the 13 top myths in this section.

Myth #1: Eating fat makes you fat

Most people believe that eating a low fat diet is critical to overcoming obesity and chronic illnesses, but in actuality, eating fat has little to do with being obese or with developing conditions such as high cholesterol hyperlipidemia, or hypertension. The fat that we eat does not turn into fat around the waist line. The fat molecules that we consume are broken down into their building blocks, which are absorbed through the mucus membranes of the intestinal tract. They have to be reconstituted and almost never do so in the same form as they were before they were broken down. Most of the fat we eat is used by the body as fuel. On the other hand, the body's own fat is built primarily from sugars and starches. The rest is used as building blocks for cell structure. (especially the essential fatty acids). Essential fatty acids do not contribute to metabolic dysfunction. In fact, they are critical for normal function of your cells and are helpful in combating metabolic problems instead of contributing to them.

Myth #2: Saturated fat contributes to obesity.

Saturated fat has very little to do with obesity. Saturated fat can and should be an important part of a healthy diet and can actually *contribute* to weight loss. Millions of people have lost weight successfully, for example, on the Atkins Diet, which contains relatively high levels of animal fat. The same applies to the Paleolithic Diet, which is becoming very popular. I am not advocating blanket use of the Atkins Diet, of course. Some people do well with it, especially Type O blood types and those with protein metabolic types. A lot of people would do well on the Atkins Diet if they limited dairy intake.

Myth #3: Eating cholesterol contributes to obesity and cardiovascular disease.

Cholesterol is a critical nutrient for human health. As a matter of fact, cholesterol is critical for the structure and function of every cell in the body. Cholesterol is the building block for sex and adrenal hormones. Moreover, it is critical for optimal brain, liver function and the repair of injured blood vessels. It is also important to note that about 85 percent of the cholesterol in your bloodstream is manufactured by your liver, so if you eat a low cholesterol or no cholesterol diet, that impacts only about 15 percent of the total cholesterol in your body. Cholesterol is critical for normal cell function and metabolism. Unfortunately, drugs like statin drugs not only lower cholesterol, but affect all of the functions that cholesterol plays a role in. The roles include mood control, brain function, muscle strength, body energy, and sexual function. This explains why taking these drugs make it harder to maintain a healthy metabolism and to be motivated to exercise and eat healthy.

Myth #4: Eggs contribute to high cholesterol and therefore contribute to sluggish metabolism.

Eggs are very high in cholesterol, specifically the egg yolk. However, as mentioned, the cholesterol you consume in food constitutes 15 percent or less of the total amount of cholesterol that is present in your body. The cholesterol in eggs contributes minimally to the cholesterol level in your blood and is helpful for increasing good cholesterol (HDL) levels and reducing bad cholesterol (LDL) levels. Eggs are also high in lecithin, a fat emulsifier, which is another healthy fat used in the body for fat transportation and normal cell function.

How your eggs are prepared is important. Certain cooking methods (hard-boiled, fried eggs that are well-done, scrambled eggs, and omelets) cause an oxidation of cholesterol in eggs, which is harmful to the body. On the other hand, healthful ways to cook eggs include those methods that keep the egg yolk runny, including soft boiled, soft poached, and fried eggs over easy fried in a healthy oil such as coconut oil or organic butter.

Myth #5: Carbohydrates are OK, but fats are not when you're trying to lose weight.

A lot of people are under the false impression that in order to lose weight, they need to follow a low fat diet, which typically means a diet high in grain-based carbohydrates. This is a recipe for weight gain—not weight loss. If the food consumed contains any refined or processed grains, they will convert to sugar and will become fat if not used for energy right away. If you want to lose weight, the best way to do so is to eat a diet that balances healthy fats with primarily low glycemic index carbohydrates and healthy proteins from organic or free range sources. In order to lose weight, the most important food groups to avoid are processed or refined carbohydrates; including breads, pastries, donuts, pasta, sweets, and candy.

Myth #6: Artificial sweeteners are better than simple sugars for weight loss.

Artificial sweeteners have little or no impact on weight. As a matter of fact, they actually increase body weight when consumed in large amounts. The reason for this is artificial sweeteners are extremely acidifying, which slows metabolism. Secondly, artificial sweeteners literally cause us to crave starches and grains more, so they often contribute to the release of insulin in response to the consumption of these sweet-tasting foods. When the insulin is released into your body, sugar levels in the bloodstream drop, causing relative hypoglycemia and cravings for starchy foods. This endless cycle, of course, contributes to more obesity and metabolic dysfunction.

Myth #7: Partially hydrogenated fats can be a healthy part of a diet.

Partially hydrogenated fats are the fats that are found in products that have long shelf lives, including packaged foods like cookies, breads, crackers, etc. Partially hydrogenated fats are also found in margarine. These fats are very harmful and affect every cell in our bodies adversely because they are incorporated as dysfunctional components of cell membranes. This causes the cell membranes to become dysfunctional and the hormone receptors on the cells stop working properly. This leads to an increased incidence of conditions such as insulin resistance and a myriad of other health challenges, including obesity.

The US Government allows a label to read, "trans-fat free" and still can contain up to 500 mg (1/2 a gram) of trans-fat which is the equivalent amount of oil in half a fish oil capsule. This can add up without even realizing that you are being exposed to these poisonous fats.

Myth #8: All animal proteins are unhealthy and disease-promoting.

The Paleolithic Diet, which was the diet of our primitive forefathers before the advent of modern civilization, was made up largely of meats, other animal proteins, fresh vegetables and fruits. There is growing evidence that some of these primitive ancestors may have had relatively long life spans (including Methuselah who was mentioned in the Bible). Our ancient ancestors didn't have grains available to them. The cultivation of grains did not start until later civilizations came along. The idea that we need grains to be healthy is simply a myth. There is more evidence and research that a diet high in animal proteins can actually be health promoting and can promote longevity. It is very clear that those who follow, for instance, the Paleolithic Diet, do very well metabolically and very seldom have problems with obesity and other obesity-related health challenges.

There are potential problems with the consumption of more meat and animal proteins, especially when consuming animals raised on genetically-engineered corn, given antibiotics and hormones as part of their raising until slaughter. This explains why some studies show that eating too much meat can be associated with diseases such as lymphoma and increased risks of cancer of the intestinal tract. However, the problem lies not with the meat or animal protein itself, but rather with what we *do* to the meat before we consume it or how we raise these animals before slaughter. The same holds true for our dairy products. Pasteurization and homogenization both have negative effects on our health and metabolism.

In our society, we see certain vicious cycles with more people suffering from stomach and digestion problems. We have epidemics of reflux, constipation, irritable bowel syndrome, inflammatory bowel disease, and cancers of the esophagus, stomach, colon, and pancreas. This is not simply because of the bad foods we are consuming, but is a result of the drugs we are using to suppress acid production in the stomach. These drugs often doom us to poor digestion, especially of high protein foods. This is another critical reason why more people have trouble consuming animal proteins such as meat. Meat that is not digested because of suppression of acid production literally will become putrefied in the intestinal tract. This greatly increases the level of toxicity in the gut, which can have adverse health effects in general.

Myth #9: Obesity is the result of too many calories in and too few calories out.

Most people believe that if you cut back on the number of calories you eat, you will lose weight. Conversely, if you burn more calories than you consume, you will lose weight.

This is a gross oversimplification.

Obesity occurs not just because of too many calories in versus calories out, but because of defective metabolisms that make it very difficult to increase our calorie burning, even when we severely restrict our calorie intake. The result is that most people who reduce their calorie intake actually slow down their metabolisms. If they do lose weight, they often lose it not because they are losing fat, but because they are losing vital lean muscle mass. Even with a marked reduction in calories, the weight will stay the same or even go up as a result of metabolism slowing down, which leads to water retention, which is another component of weight gain that is critical to understand.

If you increase your activity levels in an effort to burn more calories to lose weight and your metabolism is defective, it will be very hard for you to burn those extra calories and you will simply fall off the wagon because of an inability to maintain higher activity levels. Your body can't produce enough energy to make your metabolism run faster. Again, this is why it is critical to get to the source of the problem, which tends to be sourced at the emotional or mental level leading to adverse physical effects.

Myth #10: Low-fiber or no-fiber meals are OK.

People who drink a lot of diet drinks with no fiber in them or who eat foods that are supposedly low calorie but that contain no fiber usually end up dealing with more gastrointestinal issues like constipation. Most Americans believe they have healthy bowels if they have a bowel movement every other day, however, optimal bowel function means evacuating at least two to three times per day. We are supposed to have a built-in defecation reflex, whereby when we eat, we are supposed to move our bowels within 30 minutes to an hour after the meal (this is typically what happens to breastfed babies).

As adults, this stops happening, in part, because we actually suppress this reflex. We consume food with insufficient fiber in it or because of dysbiosis (or overgrowth of pathogenic organisms in the intestinal tract). All of these factors contribute to sub-optimal bowel function, which contributes to weight gain. In order to optimize health and metabolism, we have to optimize bowel function, and that means consuming a lot of fiber. The best way to get adequate amounts of fiber is by eating a healthy diet and avoiding diet products and diet drinks that are low in fiber. Optimizing bowel function can help you lose as much as 20 to 30 pounds, virtually overnight. That represents the amount of stool in those suffering from long-standing, severe constipation.

Myth #11: Processed foods are just as good as natural foods for maintaining and optimizing metabolism and overall health.

When we process food, we tend to corrupt it and end up turning them into disease-promoting, rather than health-promoting nutrition. Most of the diet foods on the market that people consume in order to try to lose weight are heavily processed and instead of being health-promoting are actually disease-promoting. Anytime we manipulate food in an effort to make it more palatable, make it last longer on our shelves, or make it prettier, we tend to corrupt it. The golden rule is: the fewer processed foods we consume, the better our metabolisms will be. Clean food promotes a healthier metabolism.

Myth #12: Eating fewer meals helps you lose weight.

When you eat one or two meals per day, you are much more likely to gain weight and be obese than if you eat five or six meals today. Even if you eat just as much food at each of your five or six meals as you ate during your one or two meals, your metabolism speeds up when you eat more frequently. It's a little bit like building a fire. If you want to get a fire going strong and burning tall, you use small kindling to stoke the fire rather than large, heavy logs that can stifle the fire if it's not burning very brightly. The effect of reduced frequency of meals is a slowing down of calorie burning in the body.

Myth #13: Whole grains should always be part of a healthy diet.

It is simply not true that we need grains in order to be healthy. As mentioned earlier, our forefathers ate no grains and thrived in spite of this for many thousands of years before the advent of modern agriculture. Secondly, just because something is labeled as whole grain, it does not mean that it is necessarily a true whole and unprocessed grain. If you consume grains, however, you should focus solely on authentic whole grains. But unfortunately, companies in America are allowed to use the whole grain label even when as much as 80 to 90 percent of the product is not whole grain but actually consists of processed flour!

Another reason why grains may be detrimental to your health is due to the chemicals that have been added to them. These include preservatives such as bromine, which antagonizes iodine in the human body, and trans-fatty acids, which can play havoc on your health.

Transforming Painful Exercise into Endorphin-Creating Movements

Activity is very important in managing obesity, and there is no doubt that if you want to win the battle of the bulge, you have to move—no ifs, ands, or buts about it.

There are a lot of misconceptions about exercise. Most people are confused about how to be successful at exercising. Should you do more strength training or endurance training? What forms of endurance training should you do? How much should you be exercising? Many people believe that more is better than less, but it's not always true.

In order to be successful with exercise, we need to understand the basic principles that tend to lead to success. We also need to understand why people are doing so poorly in this country with physical activity. It's not just because people are lazy. Laziness certainly is a factor, but there are reasons for this laziness or resistance to exercise. Some of these include:

- Being overwhelmed
- Stress
- Too many things to do
- Too little time
- The lack of desire to exercise
- Poor body image

We live in a society where people are overwhelmed with too much to do, too little time, and massive stress associated with the struggle to survive, to make ends meet, to feed a family, etc. Even our children are stressed out because they are overburdened with schoolwork and the social pressures to perform at higher levels. More people are being drugged, which makes it even harder for them to have healthy metabolisms. Other negative consequences of pharmaceuticals include decreased energy, increased incidence of chronic fatigue, brain fog, and other negative effects on mentation.

Our diets have a measurable impact on whether we even *want* to exercise or not. When we try inappropriate diets or inappropriate calorie restrictions, we are less likely to exercise than before. On the other hand, when you are eating healthily and taking in adequate amounts of healthy calories, you have better body and brain functions. Your body and mind actually begin to crave and enjoy exercise.

Quite a number of people sabotage themselves because of their preconceived definition of optimal exercise. In other words, if they do exercises they don't enjoy or if they have a tendency to overdo exercise when they do get to it, the likelihood of long-term success is unlikely. Even the time of day we exercise is important. People who work out in the morning, for example, are much more likely to be successful long-term than those who wait until the end of the day.

Another way to increase the likelihood of success in your efforts to exercise is to make yourself accountable to others. Tell others what you are trying to accomplish and ask them either to work out with you or to at least keep you accountable. Joining a health club often makes a difference, especially if you thrive in social environments. Others tend to be more self-conscious and introverted and do better working out on their own. Hiring a personal trainer can be a tremendous help, especially in the beginning until you have gotten into the habit and have learned how to exercise safely without risk of injury. Most people may see having a personal trainer as unaffordable, however, the short-term investment in a personal trainer once or twice a week for a month or two may be the tipping point from failure to success.

Another angle to successful exercise is to find physical activities you can enjoy and can become enthusiastic about. Hiking, biking, martial arts, or simply developing the habit of a daily walk can do wonders for your health.

Strength Training

A good strength training program is valuable in order to speed up metabolism. Strength training increases muscle mass which drives up your basal metabolic rate (which is your resting metabolic rate). Everyone should be on some form of strength training regimen if they want to improve their metabolism. Focusing on the larger muscle groups, like the stomach, the back, and the legs will do wonders. Strength training at the gym or at home 20 minutes two to three times a week is usually enough. Strength training can be done with or without sophisticated equipment. There are more and more home-based devices and DVD-based programs that involve strength training, as well as aerobics and flexibility training.

The PACE Program

There is another program that can be used by virtually anybody to speed up metabolism called the PACE program. The PACE program, or Peak 8 Program, involves doing short intervals of high level aerobic activity that lead to air hunger at the end of each short interval. Any form of aerobic exercise can be used when doing PACE. Fast walking, running or jogging, stair stepping, gliding on a glider, or even cycling can be used in this way.

PACE involves the following keys:

- Find a form of exercise that you're capable of doing, based on your health, weight, and so forth. For instance, for some it would be walking. For others who are relatively fit, jogging or cycling may be a better choice. Even arm cycling can be done for people who have very serious lower body problems or those who are paralyzed from the waist down.

- Do a warm-up period of five to ten minutes first, including stretching.

- Start your selected form of exercise, for instance, walking. Walk very rapidly for 30 to 40 seconds, making sure that by 30 to 40 seconds, you are out of breath. If you are not able to get to the point of being out of breath, it means that you need to change the form of exercise that you're doing. Add to the strenuousness of it, for example, by walking uphill instead of on level ground.

- Take a one and a half minute break in between sessions by slowing down your pace to where you are able to catch your breath.

- Repeat this process seven more times for a total of eight cycles. For those who are very unfit, six cycles may be the maximum they can achieve at first, which is fine. You can build up from there over time as your fitness level improves. You will also want to be sure to avoid injury, so if you are walking fast for 30 to 40 seconds and start feeling pains in your joints or feel like you are straining your muscles, then either change the form of exercise or be patient and work your way up to where you can do a more intense form of exercise.

- After completing your eight cycles, do a warm-down for 5 to 10 minutes. For instance, if you're walking, just slow down to an easy pace until your heart rate is back down to within 10 beats of your baseline.

First and foremost, by doing this form of exercise, we are improving metabolism tremendously with very little time spent doing exercise. Your entire exercise session should take no more than 20 minutes or 30 minutes at the most, depending on how long you warm up and warm down. It saves time, speeds up metabolism wonderfully, and has an additional benefit because it spikes human growth hormone levels. This speeds up metabolism and improves health overall, including improved cardiovascular health, heart muscle strength, and helps to build skeletal muscle (Human growth hormone is critical for the maintenance of muscle mass). This is also a great form of exercise for older individuals who have lost a lot of muscle mass because of disuse. This is a way for them to recapture that muscle mass and help them speed up their metabolisms. The spikes in human growth hormone levels also help to strengthen the immune system and recover from joint wear and tear.

In order to be able to turn our physical activity into endorphin-releasing movements, we have to dispel a number of myths that currently exist about exercise.

Myth #1: No pain, no gain. Exercise can't be fun.

This myth is entirely untrue because there are a number of things you can do that are fun, pain-free (but don't involve sitting on the couch!). The exercise that you most likely will continue with for a lifetime is going to be that activity or exercise that you enjoy. Working out to the point of pain and discomfort certainly does not equate to long-term success. Gardening, home improvement, vacuuming, cutting grass, swimming, dancing, yoga, tai chi, aerobics, mountain climbing, and sports like tennis or basketball are all great ways to have physical activity that will create plenty of endorphin releases to help spur you on to do it over and over again. You don't have to be stuck on a treadmill or walking on a track to get moving and to lose weight. Just find an activity that you enjoy doing and build it into your schedule on a regular basis.

Move, and move with a higher degree of energy.

Myth #2: It takes tremendous willpower to be successful in exercise.

It does not take tremendous willpower to consistently exercise. It only requires a shifting of your *beliefs* about exercise. All you have to do is reframe physical activity in your mind's eye in order to be successful. You may even want to consider dropping the word 'exercise' because of the negative connotation so many people have placed on this word. "Increased physical activity" may be a more useful term to use and does not come with the emotional baggage. You'll notice I seamlessly substitute the word movement for exercise. In order to make your movement/exercise work you may have to start with a clear vision of a more active you. See yourself as someone who is excited about life, is getting stronger and healthier, and able to do more fun activities. Remember, physical activity truly starts as a mental exercise rather than a physical one. Mental imaging is even used by top athletes worldwide to improve their performances. It can help you do the same. When you think like a healthy person, you tend to act like one.

Myth #3: People don't exercise because they are inherently lazy.

People who do not exercise are not necessarily lazy. They have unresolved emotional and mental conflicts that lie at the root of their sedentary lifestyle. There are some conflicts they haven't found the source of that cause them to spend more time on the couch than off the couch. A conflict of scarcity, for example, can cause someone to become a workaholic and spend all their time sitting at a desk working and trying to make ends meet, which of course negates their desire to exercise. It's the conflict of scarcity that programs for the sedentary lifestyle—not laziness. A conflict of devaluation is another example of a conflict that causes us to become couch potatoes. Because we are so self-conscious, we are reluctant to appear in public, for instance, to work out at the gym or even to take a walk down the street. For these individuals, starting at home may be the best bet or organizing workouts with others who have similar afflictions might also work. When you know and understand the conflict that has caused you to become sedentary, you are better able to create solutions and be successful as an exerciser.

Myth #4: Unless you work out hard from the beginning, you won't succeed.

The biggest mistake people make is to overdo it when they start exercising. They may feel great over the first 30 or 40 minutes but will soon realize that they are overdoing it. If they don't set a reasonable pace and schedule, they may end up causing injury or severe soreness afterwards, which may lead them to fall off the wagon again. It is much better to start slowly and build up gradually. This is critical if you want to avoid injury and muscle soreness.

Myth #5: I have too many responsibilities to have time for exercise.

One of the biggest excuses people have not to exercise regularly is time management. Time-strapped folks feel too overwhelmed and believe they can't fit another thing into their day. The truth is the more physically active you are, the more you accomplish every day and the more productive you feel, so it actually works the other way around. Overwhelm tends to be less of a problem when you incorporate physical activity into your daily life because of the increased physical energy, self-confidence, and sense of well-being. If you don't take the time for physical activity and you lose your stamina, you end up being less productive overall. This causes you to feel drained, and it adds to the vicious cycle that creates more and more stress. People who exercise regularly are simply more productive and have more energy overall when compared to people who do not get enough physical activity in their lives on a regular basis.

Myth #6: It doesn't matter what time of day you exercise.

Studies have shown that people who work out in the morning are much more likely to be successful over the long-term than those who exercise at night. Researchers followed a group of people who worked out in the morning and another group of people who worked out at night, and they discovered six months later, the people who were exercising in the morning were more likely to still be exercising than those who were trying to exercise later in the day. You generally have more energy in the morning, and exercising in the morning pumps you up for the rest of the day by giving you a nice energy boost. However, if you wait until later in the day to exercise, you do not have as much energy available, which makes it harder to convince yourself to follow through. Additionally, evening work outs tend to cause disruptions in your sleeping patterns.

Myth #7: It doesn't matter what level of priority you put exercise under.

Physical activity should be at the top of your list of priorities rather than at the bottom. If you don't put it high up on your list of priorities, then it will get swept aside and forgotten. By exercising first thing in the morning, you can mark that most important priority off your list and get on with the rest of your day while riding high on the boost of energy you received from that physical activity. As Mark Twain quipped, "If you eat a frog first thing in the morning, that will probably be the worst thing you do all day." Don't procrastinate. Get moving first thing in the morning, it may not be a replacement for coffee, but it will certainly put a spring in your step.

Myth #8: I should be strong enough to continue regular physical activity on my own without anyone else.

Accountability is very important when it comes to physical activity, and it's very difficult to hold ourselves accountable. When you have a friend who works out with you and helps you to monitor how much you do, your long-term success is much easier to achieve. In return, you get to help others and keep them accountable for their physical activity. People who have someone exercising with them on a regular basis is much more likely to stick with it because of the increased level of accountability.

Myth #9: It's OK to procrastinate on exercise.

Many people love to procrastinate because they tell themselves, "I'll start exercising at the beginning of the week." Or "My New Year's resolution will be to exercise, so I'll wait until the beginning of the year." It's important to have a plan in life, but physical activity is not something you should plan far out in the future. Get started with it today!

Cathy Bailey has lost over 20 pounds and has virtually resolved all of her symptoms related to fibromyalgia and chronic fatigue and has seen marked improvements in her overall well-being, including her emotional well-being.

###

I used to want to 'lose' fat.

After working with Dr. De Wet, I realized I don't want to 'lose' anything! I needed to gain health. I have learned to release the extra baggage (emotional) from my life and release the extra fat.

I started my effort to lose weight right after Thanksgiving 2010 and achieved my goals on all fronts by the first part of February 2011. One of the tools I used to lose the weight that I needed to was Dr. De Wet's β HCG Weight Loss Program, which starts with two days of fat loading. Thanksgiving Day came in handy as I was able to start my fat loading on that day and subsequently lost a total of 20 pounds over a period of 40 days and gained a massive amount of energy, to boot. I was trying to work on my cholesterol, and I was able to bring that down along with my weight. Also I think my general emotional well-being and self-esteem are much better.

It has been pretty easy to keep the weight off since I quit the diet. I have learned that I have to watch what I eat and simply toe the line. When my daughter was in the hospital, I gained five pounds, which was related to the stress of the serious illness that led to her hospitalization and the fact that my food options were very limited at the hospital over those few days. Of course I didn't exercise either during this time. However, I didn't feel as panicked about those five pounds as I would have in the past because I knew that I had the tools to get back where I need to be. Stress eating is still an issue, but not as bad as it was before.

Working with Dr. De Wet through Recall Healing was great because it allowed me to uncover the root causes to some lifelong issues. I was able to deal with the causes of my problems rather than just the symptoms. I found it very helpful to talk to someone who had insights that ring true and that I would not have thought about on my own. I especially appreciated the emotional support Dr. De Wet gave me.

The biggest challenge I encountered throughout my various weight loss experiences over the years revolved around days when I would eat something that wasn't healthy. My tendency was to think that I had already blown that day anyway, so I might just as well go ahead and eat whatever I wanted the rest of the day. I had to learn that it was OK to allow myself one treat, but not 15 treats. Weighing myself every single day has also been very helpful, because it helps me to stay on track with what I've accomplished and with what I am still trying to accomplish.

My habits have changed quite a bit since I lost all the weight, which has made it a lot easier for me to maintain my weight loss. I have changed my diet in such a way that I actually enjoy healthy foods a lot more now than unhealthy foods. It is a joy now to realize that those things I used to be addicted to now don't even taste good anymore. This has nothing to do with the food but has everything to do with the change of mindset.

I think while I was on Dr. De Wet's β HCG Weight Loss Program, I learned to savor every bite of food. As a matter of fact, when you are only eating 500 calories per day, you enjoy every morsel and unconscious eating tends to go by the wayside. I think that when you have the freedom to eat everything you want to eat, then you simply eat without even thinking about it, but when every single calorie that you put in your mouth matters, then you tend to pick foods you really enjoy and you savor those foods a lot more.

Chapter Seven:
We are One: Spirit-Mind-Body Connection

"You may not have the body you want, but you always have the body you need."

—Dr. Pieter De Wet

Obesity is literally analogous to a localized fat mass or can even be framed as a fatty tumor. Sometimes that fat mass covers a large area like the entire abdominal region, and sometimes it is more localized in areas such as love handles, saddle bags, double chin, and so forth. The bottom line is the fat mass, no matter where it occurs on the body, is based on a psychological emotional conflict, that programs for it. Therefore the fat mass that develops is the *result* of such a conflict. Additionally it leads to an often even bigger conflict, which we call the conflict of the diagnosis prognosis. This conflict can literally be hundreds of times more powerful than the conflict that originally programmed for obesity in the first place. Depending on the conflict program, it can program the body for a generalized increase in fat mass or sometimes it will program for an increase in fat mass in a specific area of the body. Each part of the body has a very specific meaning associated with it.

In order to resolve problems with either localized or generalized obesity permanently, we have to track down and resolve the conflict(s) programming for the disease. We can choose to explore the possibility of healing at the deepest levels, including the spiritual level. This can help us reframe who we are and allow us to discover the meaning and purpose of the fat tissue that is afflicting us.

Recall Healing refers to the concept of healing by recalling the conflict that programs for a particular disease. It is based on the principle that disease is a biological solution to an inner conflict. In order to heal from any illness, it is necessary (and often sufficient) to remove the source of conflict within oneself. Also remember that disease is the brain's best solution to keep the person alive as long as possible and is, therefore, a survival program. If you think about how the brain operates whenever we are threatened with an overwhelmingly stressful event, our subconscious mind, the automatic brain, the autonomic nervous system, and the body collude together to clear the conflict from the conscious mind. This process is described in greater detail earlier in the book. However, a couple of examples are in order to explain how it works.

The following is an example of a conflict stemming from a tragic event. When the parent of a child dies, it represents a massive shock to that child, consciously if the child is old enough or subconsciously if the child is too young to comprehend the gravity of the situation. Conversely, if a child dies, it is a massive shock to the parent. In a biological sense, when a minor trauma occurs, the conscious mind, and therefore the brain, will think it through, find a solution, and move on. In the case of a minor trauma, the brain will create a context for it and file it away without creating major ripples in the brain hemispheres.

When the conflict is so overwhelming that it cannot be put aside or worked through right away, and it can't be put into a metaphorical box in the mind, then something else *has* to happen. If you recall, the brain has a circuit breaker mechanism to prevent a blow out of your brain's 'circuitry.' When a mother loses her child, for example, she is usually so overwhelmed by that event that her brain can't think of anything else but the loss of that child. This may and often does end up incapacitating her and prevents her from responding to her environment. This prevents her from protecting herself or her other children against threats from the outside environment. This can lead to mental and physical shutdown.

In a situation like this, the brain will take whatever threatens to overwhelm it and download it to a smaller part of itself as part of a process of self-protection. An example of this is what happened to Dr. Hamer after his son was murdered when he developed a case of testicular cancer just a few months later.

Characteristics of a disease-causing conflict

Everything that happens in our bodies that is of a pathological nature is the result, at some level, of emotional conflict or high stress. Dr. Hamer discovered that the deep stress associated with his son's murder was physically downloaded to a smaller part of his brain and into his body (his testicles). Through his research, he was able to show that others suffering from testicular (and ovarian) malignancies had conflicts related to the loss of a child or even a symbolic loss. (Bankruptcy, losing a business or something that we 'nurture.')

There are four basic principles that define conflicts that cause diseases:

1. **The conflict must be dramatic.** It has to be so dramatic that it overwhelms the senses and devastates the individual to a point where it becomes difficult to take action and function normally. It can be a single, intense shock (like in Dr. Hamer's case) or it can be repetitive stresses that occur over a long period of time, such as someone who is in a bad marriage who gets beaten up every other day.

2. **The shock must be unexpected and lead to a sense of defenselessness**. The everyday stresses that we go through in life do not cause illness or obesity because we tend to anticipate them and process them effectively without them having to be downloaded. In general, we expect to be somewhat stressed in the workplace, relationships, and even financially. When additional stresses arise, it often leads to a sense of defenselessness. This can lead to the inability to communicate about theses deeply felt emotions and feelings. We can't talk to anyone about these conflicts because we feel silly or embarrassed or we feel like no one will understand us. Sometimes we feel like we don't even have time to communicate it at the time these events occur. When we fail to communicate a major stress, the brain has no other choice but to suppress it into the subconscious and into a smaller part of the brain so that the rest of the brain can be freed up for survival.

3. **The mind must be so overwhelmed that it has to download to a smaller part of itself and/or the body.** For example, with psychiatric illness, the conflict that threatens to overwhelm the brain is downloaded to a smaller part of the brain but not into the body. With generalized anxiety

disorder, depression, or schizophrenia, we have a conflict download to the brain, but not to the body. That may be the reason why people who suffer from generalized anxiety, depression, or other psychiatric illnesses are often relatively healthy otherwise. Conversely, those who live with the most physical health challenges can appear very healthy emotionally. You will often find that they cope with life very well in spite of their illnesses because they are very proficient at downloading conflicts to the body instead of just holding it in the brain.

4. **The shock leads to obsessive thoughts about what has happened.** We all have experienced situations where we just can't stop thinking about what has happened to us. Someone hurts us and we can't stop thinking about that person. We can't stop our resentment or our reflection on the hurt. We become obsessed. When the brain is threatened with overwhelm and downloads to the body, these obsessive thoughts disappear from consciousness so that we cannot find them easily or consistently. We see the conflict in the body in the form of obesity, for example, but we may find it difficult to find the conflict that *programmed* for the disease.

Most of us have no idea which conflicts are causing our diseases. They are like a blind spot or shadow in our minds. When a conflict is downloaded from the brain into the body, it disappears from our conscious mind. It stays hidden until we seek it out and discover how it is affecting our health. It is the brain and body's natural survival response to opt for short-term survival when the brain is overwhelmed by what just happened.

Whenever a conflict downloads to the body, usually you forget the details of the serious traumas that caused the disease. This would be the case of someone who survived a head on collision, someone who survived a rape, or someone who lost a loved one suddenly. You talk to them a year later, and they can hardly remember what happened even though it may be obvious that they have suffered tremendously. Often when you talk to them afterwards, they will relay the story as if it happened to someone else, almost like they are unattached to the severity of the trauma. This is because the memory of the trauma has become a blind spot in the brain.

Often those around us can see our conflicts better than we can. They may see what triggers us, for example, to overeat, stop working out, or want to go to bed instead of dealing with situations. It's not just the stress of life that programs for disease, as has been discussed before. The psychological traumas of our parents and even our genealogical roots all play a role.

The Story Behind Fat in Different Body Parts

Whenever we gain weight, the part of the body that it goes to always has something to do with the conflict that started it.

Hips and Upper Thighs (saddlebags)

The story behind fattening of the hips and/or upper thighs often relates to sexual themes. For example, when a woman is raped, fattening of the hips and/or upper thighs may be the result. Again, it is important to note that fattening may not happen immediately, but it may happen over months or years following the trauma. The initial phase following the rape when fattening has not happened yet is called the conflict active phase. This is the phase that takes place while the trauma is happening and the period following the trauma during which the mind can't let go. The way this manifests in the body called the "conflict active phase." During this phase there is thinning that takes place in the fat tissue in the body part that the brain links to the trauma physically or symbolically. For instance, at the time of the trauma, there is no obesity. When that same individual, for instance, enters a romantic relationship at a later date, the brain will activate the fattening program in this particular area of the body, causing a fattening of the hips and upper thighs. This happens during the recovery phase.

For details on the different phases of disease and other details about how conflicts program for disease, get my other book, *Heal Thyself: Transform Your Life, Transform Your Health*

It is as if the body prepares itself to protect against further violations by fortifying the entry point involved in this previous trauma, which occurred around the pelvic region. The subconscious program also may have something to do with making the individual less of a target by making that body part involved in the trauma less attractive.

Fat on the inside of the upper thighs is often linked to a story of molestation, rape, or other painful sexual themes. The hips, on the other hand, are associated with fertility-related themes. Paradoxically, the fattening on the outside of the hips often emphasizes the fact that a woman is highly fertile. It can also be linked to a biological program directed towards a male suitor by overemphasizing a display of fertility.

The thighs can become even more prominent if there is a memory of some drama related to the delivery of a baby. For example, a woman who had a difficult delivery in which the baby died may develop larger thighs. Sometimes it can be genealogical as well, which means she is carrying an epigenetic memory of a difficult delivery or the loss of an infant at birth in a previous generation.

Outer Thighs

Fattening of the outer thighs is often a sign of anger, especially anger toward the opposite sex. The outside of the hips is associated with the gallbladder meridian, which is related to resentment and anger, especially within the family or a symbolic family. When you see someone with big outer thighs, it's usually a reflection of some kind of anger or resentment going on within their family.

Upper and Lower Legs

In Recall Healing we relate the legs in general to our actual or symbolic mother (arms to actual or symbolic father). Often you will find that women who have thick legs were abandoned or felt abandoned by their mothers (this abandonment could be real, imaginary, virtual, or symbolic). Even when the trauma was not perpetrated by the mother, in the case of incest, the victim feels symbolically abandoned by the mother because the mother did not protect the child. In a parallel fashion, perhaps there is a subconscious belief that she did not take good enough care of the father who perpetrated the molestation. This has nothing to do with reality (or logic): it is simply what the subconscious mind programs for as a consequence of this kind of trauma.

Outside of Upper Thighs

With saddle bags or fattening of the upper thighs usually there is a memory related to abandonment by the father. The 'saddlebags' could be storage sites linked to protection against famine and starvation. If I am abandoned by my father as a child, my biological brain will add weight to this area as a method to increase the energy reserves on hand because I have to stand 'alone' without my father's support. If there is a history of famine in the family or in a previous generation, there is an epigenetic imprint for the body to store up energy supplies as reserves. (i.e. if a family went through the Great Depression and someone almost starved to death or if the family lost everything) If your mother is deprived of food or something symbolic of food, for example, while she is pregnant, that can cause prominent saddle bags to develop in you. If the father is compensating for a weak mother, (if the father had to be the mother as well as the father) then you will often see saddle bags develop in his female children later on.

Double Chin

Someone who has a double chin tends to have had a trauma that relates to being forced to live a double life, hence, the term we use when we say that someone is two-faced. They have one face that they show to the world, and another face that they show to people who are close to them. If someone has three chins, the biological meaning is being three-faced.

For example, when you look at a picture of Alfred Hitchcock, he had three chins and led three lives. In his first life, he was a happily married man who took care of his family. His second life, as a movie director, was very complex. He made movies with interesting and elaborate stories. In his third life, he had a very complex inner emotional world in which he wrote all kinds of weird and wonderful stories. In short, Hitchcock was a warm family man, an extroverted movie maker, and a creative and introverted writer.

Usually people who have a double or triple chin will go to extraordinary lengths to protect their privacy. It's again, like living two lives, which generally means that they are hiding something from the outside world, from their family, or both. This secrecy is linked to a devaluation that they feel or some secret that is hidden just beneath the surface. This is not to insinuate that people with double chins are purposefully keeping secrets from the world, but in many cases there is a theme of secrecy linked to devaluation or even a conflict of separation involved.

Lower Abdomen

If the lower part of the abdomen is obese, we may see that there is an element of deep insecurity and devaluation. Lower abdominal obesity also is often linked to real or symbolic abandonment by the mother or a conflict of separation associated with the mother. When we have more fattening of the upper abdomen, there tends to be an element of self-protection. For example, if a person has to be more menacing in order to protect oneself or the family, the biological brain might be programming them to become a wedge between their parents. (i.e. a child who grows up around physical abuse in the family) If there is a conflict of separation from or abandonment by the father, the upper abdomen will tend to become the target organ. Interestingly enough, if a child or adult is traumatized in the abdominal region, (i.e. if he were kicked in the stomach by a horse when he was growing up) there may be a generalized increase in fat in the upper and lower abdomen. The same also applies to someone who has gone through surgery and was traumatized by the surgeon's knife.

Notch in the Mid-Hip Area

A notch in the mid-hip area is rather strange phenomenon that happens with many women. They often have prominent hips with a big dent below the hip area, followed by prominent saddle bags lower on the hips. When this notch occurs, it is usually linked to a conflict connected to unwanted intimacy with a man that they are close to or who is constantly present in their environment. For example, if a woman is married and for some reason feels estranged from her husband and does not want intimacy or affection from him, but she's conflicted by that, there may be a notch in this section of the thigh. The section of the hip where the dent occurs above the thigh and below the hip is called the trochanter. This area corresponds to themes related to marriage, home, motherhood, and maternity.

Buttocks

Prominent buttocks, like prominent hips, often reflects a deep subconscious desire to attract a man. When the buttocks are very large, there is usually some kind of trauma of abandonment by a male, either the father or a symbol of the father, such as a male relationship or male partner. It's no accident that large buttocks often are paired with large breasts in most women. Large breasts serve the same purpose of attracting a male partner. Enlargement in this area anthropologically symbolizes fertility.

On the other hand, women with small hips and small buttocks, often have the conflict of not wanting to attract attention. If there is a sexual trauma in the family, (rape, incest, or sexual violation of any kind) in proceeding generations, a woman may have more masculine characteristics (small buttocks, small hips, and less prominent breasts). Strange as it may seem, if the father desperately wanted a boy and not a girl, the newborn girl may take on the shape of a boy more than a girl. This is prominent in Eastern cultures where great emphasis is placed on having boys rather than girls and sadly, where infanticide of female infants is not uncommon.

Cellulite

The development of cellulite has to do with the need for protection. With cellulite, there is often an element of fear: fear of loss, fear of losing security, your home, or any protection. For example, if a woman's husband has an affair or she fears that her husband will leave her (fear of abandonment), she will often develop cellulite in response to the fear of losing her security or home. Cellulite often develops on the part of the body that corresponds best with a particular conflict, so if the cellulite is more on the buttocks, often there is an element of feeling rejected sexually. On the other hand, if it's on the sides of the thighs, often there is an element of needing to protect oneself because of fear for ones' survival. When the conflict is resolved the cellulite will tend to disappear.

Often cellulite can also be linked to a woman not wanting her husband's affections, so the cellulite is symbolic of her trying to protect herself from her husband, who she feels has violated her in some way. Cellulite involves swelling and thickening of the skin. Cellulite of the legs might occur in the case of women who have children who leave the 'nest' early. In this case, a conflict arises when the mother refuses to emotionally let her child go. Cellulite can also develop as a form of protection because of the fear of not having the mother's protection, agreement, or love.

Very large upper and lower legs combined with cellulite

Some women have very fat lower legs and thighs with an excess amount of cellulite. This is called the mermaid syndrome. When a mother is holding a daughter back and not allowing her to live her life by leaving the nest (or resents her for leaving the nest) the daughter may develop legs that are big from top to bottom. On the other hand, if the legs are big between the ankles and knees but nowhere else, one may have a conflict related to not having a mother's approval. If our efforts to gain approval is rejected, the conflict programs will result in increased fat storage in that area.

Releasing Your Inner Demons and Letting Spirit Guide Your Healing

There are dozens of example of physical, emotional and belief-centered tactics for *Bringing Sexy Back*, if you want to distill all of these pages into a single strategy, this is it! Below are three keys to healing any conflict that programs for diseases including obesity:

1. Name it.

2. Claim it.

3. Dump it.

The first step in healing obesity or any other disease is to be able to name the conflict programming for your disease. However, more important than naming your conflict is *laying* claim to it. I call this healing through revelation. A revelation is an insight that is so powerful that it can change the course of a disease and may even lead to miraculous healing.

Name It

Naming the conflict is, at best, an academic exercise that gives you some insight into the reasons why you have developed a certain problem. Claiming your conflict means that you have gained massive insight that makes the dumping of it much more likely and achievable. Every disease, including obesity, contains insights within it that represent the gift or the blessing that a disease process bestows upon you. Through studying your diseases and afflictions, you get to learn a great deal about yourself, your project purpose, and your genealogy. You also learn the ultimate truth about obesity and your body in general. The big, bold truth is, you may not have the body that you want, but you always have the body you need.

Naming the conflicts programming for our diseases begin with understanding each disease and associating the common conflicts that can program for it. Learning a little bit about your physiology and what happens during the two phases of disease creation (conflict active and conflict resolution phase) helps us to understand our symptoms better. It also makes it easier to map where we are in the disease process. For example, when we look at obesity, our process of healing starts with being able to name the conflicts programming for our obesity. Being able to name our conflicts means becoming knowledgeable about all the programs that can trigger obesity. There are distinct steps one should take. Here they are in order of importance:

1. Know your life's story.
2. Learn about what happened while you were in the womb.
3. Seek details on your genealogy.

Start a journal, jotting down what you can recall about your personal life and all of your experiences. Memories of certain traumatic events will surface. This will give you a better understanding of your conflicts programming your disease.

Ask your parents, if they are alive, what happened to them while your mother was pregnant with you. Finding out the details of their life, feelings and circumstances will be interesting and revealing.

Get as much personal and experiential information about your grandparents, great-grandparents and beyond. The more you understand their lives and stories, the clearer the epigenetic tapestry will be uncovered.

Interestingly enough, about 10 percent of people are able to cure their illnesses, including conditions such as obesity, simply by being able to *name* the conflicts programming for the illness.

Claim It

After you name the conflict programming for your disease, the process of claiming it begins. That process involves remembering what exactly happened to you just before the disease started. For example, if you started becoming overweight at the age of 20 years and one month, we want to know what trauma immediately preceded that event. Sometimes we find a single traumatic event, and other times we will find a series of smaller traumatic events leading up to the process of weight gain. Then dig into the exact emotions that we *felt* at the time as we were going through those life events or traumas. In other words, we are literally gaining access to the program that is causing the obesity and getting to reprocess the emotions attached to the traumatic experiences leading up to the weight gain. This process allows us to cry the tears that were never cried, to release the fears that were never released, to gain the empathy and comfort that were never gained, and to revalue ourselves if we felt devalued. Up to fifty percent of patients are able to resolve their disease process, including obesity, with these first two steps. That bears restating.

Up to 50% of patients are able to release their obesity by clearly allowing themselves to non-judgmentally recall their feelings during a past conflict.

In fact, this process often leads to a spontaneous dumping, especially if circumstances have changed and the traumas that were suffered at the time are not present anymore. For example, if a woman started becoming obese while in a very troubled marriage, in which she was physically abused, she may be able to dump the conflict a lot easier if she is not in that relationship anymore and has moved on. On the other hand, if she is still in that troubled marriage and continually being physically abused, the dumping process might be more difficult to achieve.

Dump It

The dumping process involves one of two steps: either repairing or reframing. In the example just given, a woman who is in an abusive relationship can repair the situation by either getting out of the relationship or by going to counseling with her husband if he is willing to do so. On the other hand, if she is not willing to separate and if her husband refuses to attend counseling with her, the only option available to her is to reframe. The repair of a conflict and the reframe of a conflict both involve communication. We have to talk about our conflicts and traumas to someone who can listen to us without judgment or attachments. This is best done with a skilled professional or enlightened mentor: otherwise it will be difficult for them to hear our stories. It could be your best friend, counselor, teacher, or a healthcare provider, but we have to be able to communicate the details of what happened and the experience as it was actually felt, not what we think we should have felt. The 50 percent of people who are unsuccessful in clearing their conflict through the naming and claiming process have to go through this third phase, which involves dumping the conflict. There are a number of useful tools that can help us dump our conflicts and traumas. Here are some of the most common tools:

1. Emotional Freedom Technique (EFT): combines the tapping on acupressure points on the body with psychological tools involving the naming of the problem and then the naming of the solution. For further information on EFT, visit www.qhiwellness.com.

2. Neuro-linguistic programming (NLP): involves the reprogramming of the subconscious.

3. Journey work: From the book *The Journey* by Brandon Bays. In her book, she describes a process of being able to simulate a communication with someone who has traumatized you or who has been lost, even if they have

died. In your mind's eye, you can have this conversation with someone to clear yourself of the wound you are dealing with.

4. Hypnosis, commonly used in the field of Recall Healing.

5. Timeline therapy: allows you to go back to the traumatic experiences of your life and literally change the context of the experience by changing how you feel about it now looking back at it in a different light. This therapy is often done in conjunction with hypnosis.

6. *Ho'oponopono* exercise: a Hawaiian healing technique that revolves around creating an apology and an affirmation that leads to the release of deep-seated traumas. It gives you the ability to take ownership of your hurts and traumas instead of waiting for others to apologize. *Ho'oponopono* involves the recognition that all of us are responsible in some way for the traumas and hurts that we've experienced in life and the fact that every relationship represents a two-way street. For instance, we often blame the parents for traumatizing the baby but fail to recognize that the baby coming into this world also represents a trauma to the parents at some level, even though that trauma was not caused on purpose.

In this light of recognition, we are able to make the statement "I am sorry" to virtually anyone, including our parents. This leads us to the next step, which is to ask for forgiveness by saying "Please forgive me".

When you ask for forgiveness it allows you to move on with your life.

The next step in *Ho'oponopono* is to say "Thank you." The "Thank you" is a recognition that even the traumas that affected you somehow contributed to your life in a positive way. Remember that you can be blessed by adversity just as much as you can be blessed by the good deeds of others. The "thank you" recognizes the lessons you've learned through your experience. There is always a silver lining, always something good that comes from every situation.

The final step is to say "I love you." Say this (either in your mind's eye or directly to those who have touched your life), even if that impact was primarily traumatic and it will empower you. *Ho'oponopono's* power lies in its ability to help us be able to truly forgive at the deepest level.

7. My heart is full of love and understanding: This exercise involves putting your left hand over your heart with your right hand over your left hand. Then you make the statement, "My heart is full of love and understanding." You repeat that over and over for about a minute or two or until you feel a warm sensation in your chest. Then you say that the other person's heart is full of love and understanding. Just insert the name of the person who's causing you conflict, and say "their heart is full of love and understanding" until you feel a warm sensation in your chest.

8. Butterfly hug: This exercise involves giving yourself a hug by placing your left hand on your right upper arm and your right hand on your left upper arm and patting yourself, alternating with the left and right hand. This can be combined with a statement such as, "even though I have this deep 'emotion' (for example anger), towards this 'person' (for example, my spouse), I refuse to be tormented

by this for the rest of my life and it is in my best interests to let this 'emotion' (for example, anger), go now. I refuse to let this 'emotion' (anger) that I've been holding onto continue to make me sick, either physically or emotionally.

My Own Story

One of the questions we should always ask when affected by obesity is what happened just before you started becoming overweight. For example, when I was in my late 30s I went through a very painful divorce. My first marriage had a lot of ups and downs and was pretty volatile. At the beginning of the relationship that led to that marriage, I had no problems with obesity or weight.

Like many young couples, I went through a semi-traumatic courting experience, and then ended up marrying my first wife. But by the time I got married, my weight had escalated from about 154 pounds to about 164 pounds in the two years preceding my marriage.

After my first year of marriage my weight continued to increase because of my conflicts. The major one was a survival conflict when I emigrated from South Africa to the USA.

I left everything behind when I left South Africa and had a distinct survival conflict. I arrived with scarce resources and a massive responsibility: a wife, a three-month-old child, six suitcases, and a couple thousand dollars in my pocket. It was sink or swim for me, as a result because of this stress, I lost much of my weight, dropping down into the low 150's.

My weight finally stabilized when I got to a place where I was more comfortable with my career. I was studying holistic medicine at the time and my weight began to gradually rise. By the time my marriage to my first wife ended, I was 37 years old and my body weight had increased to 176 pounds. Additional education while practicing emergency medicine compounded the stress. I was committed to introduce holistic concepts to the university setting where I taught academic medicine as a family physician. This became a very stressful endeavor with only token support from the bureaucracy that I was working under. The fat kept adding up. Add in a divorce and you can see that my body needed protection!

When I started dating, (my soon-to-be second wife) my weight actually decreased all the way down to 162 pounds until we got married. When I got married for the second time at the end of 1998, life became a bit more complicated again as my wife and I took on the challenges of blending our families, working together to practice integrative medicine in a part of the country where this kind of medicine was almost unheard of! (Northeast Texas)

My stress was about to go into overdrive. First, I started a new practice in an area where the awareness about holistic medicine was limited. Next, I incurred all the financial stress of a new practice. On top of that, I had the consequences of daily stress from going through my divorce from my first wife. With this trifecta of stress, you can understand why my weight started going up again. During and following this time, my weight escalated again into the 180's.

It was about to get worse.

In 2004, I became the target of the established medical establishment due to the style of medicine I practiced. As a result, my weight escalated from the 180's to 192 pounds. I was legally and morally attacked by the system and ended up spending insane amounts of money to defend myself. My weight continued to escalate into the 200's. When my weight reached 204 pounds, I surrendered a secret habit I had taken on when I first got married and when I was finishing medical school, believe it or not.

I was a closet smoker for many years until 2010.

When I quit smoking, my weight escalated even more and eventually settled at portly 215 pounds. No matter what I did, I could not shed the weight. In 2010, I started following the β HCG weight loss program that I had customized for my patients.

I lost 40 pounds in 40 days.

As part of my β HCG program, we teach patients to address the emotional roots of their obesity, which is exactly what I did for myself. I was my own guinea pig. Not only did the β HCG do the trick, but by using the conflict resolution strategies in this book, I was able to effortlessly stop smoking forever. This didn't happen overnight, of course.

Even though I had been doing Recall Healing work with patients for over seven years with great success, I had difficulty doing my own work in isolation. By mustering up the courage to involve my mentors and teachers, together we got to the roots of these health challenges and addictions. I did exactly what I teach, which is to:

1. Name it
2. Claim it
3. Dump it

It is truly that simple. I succeeded only with the knowledge outlined in this book (and others), the commitment to become more self-aware and the support of those people who cared about me and mattered in my life.

Whenever you are dealing with obesity or any kind of chronic illness, it is critical to track down the underlying conflicts programming for the condition and to resolve or reframe them. There are many tools available to access and clear these conflicts. Recall Healing, in my experience, is the best way to access the subconscious where most of these programming and triggering conflicts of disease are hidden. With obesity, it is critical to go back, look at what you were going through in your life just prior to your weight escalations. On occasion you will not find anything in your life, but when you look at your genealogy, you will find something. It could be an event or events that happened to your ancestors, your parents or you. Take a look at your history, your family history, ask the right questions and learn to let go, of that which does not serve you anymore. The more you seek, the more you will find.

When dealing with chronic illness of any kind it is important to discover the program that your body is running to resolve the conflict that underlies that program. If you can't uncover the program, you will never be able to truly heal from obesity. Your body is your guide as you take this journey of self-discovery. By understanding the programs and conflicts that resulted in your weight gain, you can pinpoint exactly what caused you to gain the weight, even if you were completely unaware of these conflicts previously. Your body reads like a textbook. Every single symptom and condition is a piece of the puzzle. Obesity is easily solved once you decipher the clues and understand why you are the way that you are. There is always a solution, but you have to follow the clues and unlock the answer.

If you don't see anything in your own life that could possibly be causing a conflict that leads to obesity, it is important to look at the lives of your parents, especially right before, during, and after your conception and birth. This period of time is called your project purpose, which directly affects you even at a physical level, even before you were born. You may have no idea what even happened to them, and yet you are still deeply affected by their experiences. If you are unable to discover anything significant related to your project purpose, then your investigation needs to extend beyond that period of time to other parts of your genealogy. Go back at least three generations, if possible. You never know exactly what you will find, but if you go deep enough you will almost always find a connection between what is happening to your body now and what happened in past generations.

These genealogical downloads are very important because unresolved conflicts tend to get passed down from generation to generation. This is why obesity and other chronic illnesses tend to run in families. It may have very little to do with genetics. These unresolved conflicts keep getting passed down from generation to generation until someone in the family does something to resolve these conflicts, not just for themselves, but also on behalf of the family. For further clues on genealogical aspects that might be contributing to your problems with obesity, look especially at those in your family tree who align with birth order. Also look at family secrets, deep traumas that were suffered by your ancestors, including unexpected losses, and even family curses.

Conflicts can be cleared in one of three ways. They can be resolved by finding specific solutions, some of which we have discussed previously in this book, or we can take positive action to reframe the conflict in order to neutralize it. A third option is to transcend a conflict through love, compassion, insight, awareness, or by finding a spiritual framework.

Of course a critical and helpful component is adding healthy nutrition, exercise, and other important lifestyle changes. These strategies make it easier to increase your mental and physical energies, transform your health and lose weight permanently.

The Spiritual Connection

There is a spiritual part of healing and weight loss that must be understood. When we talked about the five levels of healing, we mentioned that the fifth level has to do with the spirit body, which is influenced profoundly by religious and spiritual pursuits. Tools such as prayer and meditation tend to be very helpful. This is also the realm where empowering rituals, whether spiritually or religiously based, can help bring about dramatic healing. In fact, the spirit body has the greatest potential to be the catalyst for miracles to occur. However, we need to realize that certain religious beliefs can also create massive unintentional *obstacles* for healing.

If those religious beliefs contribute to the accumulation of negative emotions, such as guilt, shame, fear, anger, or any other disempowering emotions, it will create an unstoppable block to healing. There are some religious institutions who control their flock through fear and intimidation. When an institution promulgates ideas that members should believe a certain way and tithe a certain amount or risk everlasting damnation, they are deriving undue influence and control. These emotions and beliefs are represented through the bottom half of the map of consciousness as represented in David Hawkin's book *Power Versus Force*. The bottom half of the map represents consciousness doesn't lead to healing. The more we are trapped in the 8 negative emotions and associated beliefs represented on the lower section of the map of consciousness the less likely we are to heal. Those 8 emotions are:

1. Shame

2. Guilt
3. Apathy
4. Grief
5. Fear
6. Desire
7. Anger
8. Pride

When we hold disempowering belief systems, whether religious-based or otherwise, it makes healing from anything very difficult, especially from chronic illnesses. For example, a lot of people dealing with morbid obesity have a deep-seated belief that their condition is deserved as a punishment from God. They often have a deep-seated belief that they are undeserving of healing. Sixty percent of patients I see have a core spiritual conflict related to deserving good health and are therefore blocked from healing. In essence, there is a real wall preventing them from long-term or profound healing. In order to heal, we have to understand that it's not God's will for us to be sick. It is God's will for us to be as healthy as we can be and for us to heal. When you understand disease at the level of the spiritual realm and based on Recall Healing principles discussed throughout this book, we can know that a disease is a biological solution. It is simply the brain's best method for keeping us alive as long as possible. Therefore, disease is a survival program, and by extension, a *blessing* from God.

We mentioned earlier when discussing the map of consciousness that the way we see our Creator is directly correlated with the way we see ourselves and the way we look at the world. For example, people who believe that God is a judgmental, wrathful God experience themselves in the same way—as judgmental and wrathful. This tends to be the way they act towards others.

On the other hand, people who see God as an unconditionally loving being who is wise, forgiving, and merciful, will feel and act wise, forgiving and merciful. It is obvious which of these two beliefs is more likely to allow healing to occur. It is critical to learn to move beyond self-judgment, forgive ourselves unconditionally, and forgive others unconditionally in order to heal. This means that we ought to look at our creator in the same light as a God of unconditional forgiveness.

Remember, you were created in God's image and likeness, which means that you were patterned after God's own divinity. Discover that within yourself and you've just taken a huge step towards healing.

In your service,

Pieter De Wet, M.D.

Quantum Healing Institute & Tyler Total Wellness Center
212 Old Grande Blvd., Ste C114 Tyler, Texas 75703

Direct: 903.939.2069
Toll Free: 877.484.9735
Email: info@QHIWellness.com
http://www.qhiwellness.com

Bibliography

Bays, Brandon, *The Journey,* NY: Simon and Schuster, 1999.

Benor, Daniel, J. MD. *Spiritual healing, scientific validation of a healing revolution.* Southfield, MI: Vision Publications, 1992

Chopra, Deepak, MD, *Quantum healing: exploring the frontiers of mind-body medicine*, NY: Bantam Books, 1989

Christiano, Joseph. *Blood Types, Body Types and You.* Lake Mary, FL: Siloam Press, 2000.

Colbert, Don, MD. *Deadly Emotions: Understand the Mind-Body-Spirit Connection That Can Heal or Destroy You.* Nashville, Thomas Nelson, Inc., 2003 — *The Seven Pillars of Health.* Lake Mary, FL: Siloam Press, 2007.

Cowden, W. Lee, MD; Ferry Akbar Pour, MD; Russ Dicarlo; and Burton Golberg. *Longevity: An Alternative Medicine Definitive Guide.* Tuburon, CA: Alternative Medicine Books, 2001.

D'Adamo, Dr. Peter J. and Catherine Whitney. *Eat Right 4 Your Type.* New York: J. P. Putnam's Sons,1996.

De Wet, Pieter, *Heal Thyself,* Mustang, OK: Tate Publishing 2010.

Finely, Guy, *Designing your own destiny*, Llewellyn Publications, 1995

Ford, Debbie. *The Secret of the Shadow: The Power of Owning Your Whole Story.* New York: Harper Collins Publishers, Inc., 2002 —*The dark side of the light chasers,* New York: Riverhead Books, Berkeley Publishing Group, 1998

Fromm, Erich. *To Have or to Be? A New Blueprint for Mankind.*

London: Abacus, 1976.

Galland, Leo, MD. *The Four Pillars of Healing: How the New Integrated Medicine Can Cure You.* New York: Random House, Inc., 1997.

Hamer. Reiki—Dramatic New Medicine Disease Chart.

Hawkins, David R., MD, PhD. *Power vs. Force: The Hidden Determinants of Human Behavior.* Carlsbad, CA: Hay House, Inc., 2002.

Hay, Louise L. *You Can Heal Your Life.* Carlsbad, CA: Hay House, Inc., 1999.

Hyman, Mark, MD. *Ultra-Metabolism: The Simple Plan for Automatic Weight Loss.* New York: Scribner, 2006.

Mercola, Joseph MD, Dr. *Mercola's Total Health program,* Schaumburg, IL: Mercola.com 2003-2006

Michaels, Jillian, *Master your metabolism,* New York: Crown Publishers, 2009

Myss, Caroline PHD, *Why people don't heal and how they can,* New York: Three Rivers Press, Crown Publishers, 1997

Obissier, Patrick. *Biogenealogy: Decoding the Psychic Roots of Illness.* Rochester, VT: Healing Arts Press, 2006.

Padus, Emrika. *The Complete Guide to Your Emotions & Your Health: New Dimensions in Mind/Body Healing.* Emmaus, PA: Rodale Press, Inc., 1986.

Renaud, Gilbert, PhD., *Recall Healing: Unlocking the Secrets of Illness — Eating Disorders: Obesity, Bulimia, Anorexia and Other Digestive Related Disorders—Pyramid of Health,* Self-published by Gilbert Renaud and Total Biology Consulting.

Schutzenberger, Anne A. *The Ancestor Syndrome: Transgenerational Psychotherapy and the Hidden Links in the Family Tree.* Hove, East Sussex: Routledge, 2007.

Truman, Karol K. *Feelings Buried Alive Never Die.* St. George, UT: Olympus Distributing, 2003.

Wright, Henry W. *A More Excellent Way: Be in Health.* Thomaston, GA: Pleasant Valley Publications, 2005.

Young, Robert O., PhD. and Shelley Redford Young. *The pH Miracle: Balance Your Diet, Reclaim Your Health.* New York: Wellness Central–Hachette Book Group, 2002— *The pH Miracle for Weight Loss: Balance Your Body Chemistry, Achieve Your Ideal Weight.* New York: Wellness Central–Hachette Book Group, 2005.

Made in the USA
San Bernardino, CA
21 February 2015